NURSING FACULTY SECRETS

LINDA J. SCHEETZ, EdD, RN, CS, CEN

Professor and Chair
Division of Nursing
Mount Saint Mary College
Newburgh, New York

HANLEY & BELFUS, INC./Philadelphia

Publisher: HANLEY & BELFUS, INC.
                  Medical Publishers
                  210 South 13th Street
                  Philadelphia, PA 19107
                  (215) 546-7293; 800-962-1892
                  FAX (215) 790-9330
                  Web site: http://www.hanleyandbelfus.com

Disclaimer: This book is not intended to be prescriptive, but rather offers the collective wisdom of nursing faculty. Although the information in the book has been carefully reviewed for accuracy, neither the authors nor the editor nor the publisher can accept any legal responsibility for any errors. Neither the publisher nor the editor makes any warranty, expressed or implied, with respect to the material contained herein. Case studies are profiled from the collective experiences of nurse faculty. Names and other identifying information have been changed to protect anonymity.

Library of Congress Cataloging-in-Publication Data

Scheetz, Linda Jean.
     Nursing faculty secrets/Linda J. Scheetz.
        p.;cm.—(The Secrets Series®)
     Includes bibliographical references and index.
     ISBN 1-56053-423-0 (alk. paper)
        1. Nurses—Employment—Examinations, questions, etc. 2. Nurses—
     Selection and appointment—Examinations, questions, etc. 3. Nursing
     schools—Faculty—Examinations, questions, etc. 4. Nurses—Study and
     teaching—Examinations, questions, etc. I. Title. II. Series.
        [DNLM: 1. Faculty, Nursing—Examination Questions. 2. Education,
     Nursing—Examination Questions. WY 18.2 S315n 2000]
     RT73 .S295 2000
     610.73'071'1—dc21
                                                        00-037044

NURSING FACULTY SECRETS   ISBN 1-56053-423-0

Last digit is the print number: 9   8   7   6   5   4   3   2   1

CONTENTS

I. HIGHER EDUCATION AND THE FACULTY ROLE

1. Landing That Faculty Position: A View from Both Sides   1
   Linda S. Smith, DSN, RN

2. Gaining Perspective: Organizational Structure   9
   Mary Lou Rusin, EdD, RN

3. The Role of Faculty Within the College or University.   14
   Elizabeth N. Stokes, EdD, RN, and Christine M. Henshaw, MN, RN

II. THE SACRED TRIAD: TEACHING, RESEARCH, AND SERVICE

4. Classroom Teaching   25
   Sister Leona DeBoer, PhD, RN

5. Clinical Teaching   38
   Priscilla L. Sagar, EdD, RN

6. Research and Scholarship.   49
   Dolores A. Bower, PhD, RN, and Bernadette D. Curry, PhD, RN

7. Faculty Service Activities.   53
   Victoria Rizzo Nikou, PhD, RN, CS

8. Academic Advisement   57
   Sandra Y. Barnes, PhD, RN

III. NEGOTIATING THE SYSTEM

9. Faculty Workload   61
   Dolores A. Bower, PhD, RN, and Vicki Smith, MSN, RN

10. Faculty Evaluation   64
    Dolores A. Bower, PhD, RN, and Ann H. Venuto, MS, RN

11. Mentoring New Faculty   68
    Anita L. Throwe, MS, RN, CS, and Sandra B. Weatherford, MSN, RN, FNP, CEN

12. Preparing for Tenure.   74
    Anne Manton, PhD, RN, CEN

IV. ISSUES AND TEACHING STRATEGIES IN NURSING EDUCATION

13. Legal and Ethical Issues.   81
    Christine M. Henshaw, RN, MN, and Linda J. Scheetz, EdD, RN, CS, CEN

14. Concerns of and about Students   90
    *Elizabeth N. Stokes, PhD, RN, Geraldine Valencia-Go, PhD, RN, CS, and
    Kelly Fisher, MS, RN*

15. Students with Special Needs. 102
    Linda J. Allan Pasto, MS, RN, and Geraldine Valencia-Go, PhD, RN, CS

16. Student Evaluation 112
    Linda J. Scheetz, EdD, RN, CS, CEN

17. Teaching to a Diverse Student Group: Transcultural Concepts 123
    Linda S. Smith, DSN, RN

18. The Learning Resource Center. 130
    Kelly L. Fisher, MS, RN

19. Integrating Technology in the Classroom. 136
    Gail K. Baumlein, PhD(c), RN, CNS

20. Curriculum Development 140
    Beth Davies, EdD, RN

21. Teaching and Evaluating Critical Thinking 147
    Ann M. Gothler, PhD, RN

22. Developing Written Assignments. 155
    Ann M. Gothler, PhD, RN

V. ON THE HORIZON

23. The New Millennium: The Role of Distance Education 161
    Carla Mueller, PhD(c), RN

24. Organizational Membership and Political Education: Our Future is Now. 168
    Elizabeth A. Mahoney, EdD, ACRN

VI. PULLING IT ALL TOGETHER

25. Lessons Learned: Perspectives from a New Faculty Member 177
    Jenny Radsma, MN, RN

26. Been There, Done That: Case Studies in Nursing Education. 183

INDEX 191

CONTRIBUTORS

Sandra Y. Barnes, PhD, RN
Associate Professor, Department of Nursing, Chicago State University, College of Health Sciences, Chicago, Illinois

Gail K. Baumlein, PhD(c), RN, MSN
Instructor, Med Central Health System School of Nursing, Mansfield, Ohio

Dolores A. Bower, PhD, RN
Dean and Professor, College of Nursing, Niagara University, Niagara, New York

Bernadette D. Curry, PhD, RN
Associate Professor, College of Nursing, Niagara University, Niagara, New York

Beth H. Davies, EdD, RN
Assistant Professor, Division of Nursing, Mount Saint Mary College, Newburgh, New York

Sister Leona DeBoer, PhD, RN
Professor of Nursing and Coordinator of the Graduate Program, Division of Nursing, Mount Saint Mary College, Newburgh, New York

Kelly L. Fisher, MSN, RN
Assistant Professor, Undergraduate Department of Nursing, Simmons College, Boston, Massachusetts

Ann M. Gothler, PhD, RN
Professor and Chair, Division of Nursing, The Sage Colleges, Troy, New York

Christine M. Henshaw, MN, RN
Instructor, Department of Nursing, Highline Community College, Des Moines, Washington

Elizabeth Anne Mahoney, EdD, MS, ACRN
Professor, Division of Nursing, The Sage Colleges, Troy, New York

Anne P. Manton, PhD, RN, CEN
Associate Professor and Acting Dean, School of Nursing, Fairfield University, Fairfield, Connecticut

Carla Mueller, PhD(c), RN
Associate Professor and Director of Instructional Technology, Departments of Nursing and Allied Health, University of Saint Francis, Fort Wayne, Indiana

Victoria Rizzo Nikou, PhD, RN, CS
Assistant Professor, Hunter-Bellevue School of Nursing, Hunter College of the City University of New York, New York, New York

Linda Allen Pasto, MS, RN
Professor, Department of Nursing, Tompkins-Cortland Community College, Dryden, New York

Jenny Radsma, RN, MN
Assistant Professor, Division of Nursing, University of Maine at Fort Kent, Fort Kent, Maine

Mary Lou Rusin, EdD, RN
Professor and Chair, Department of Nursing, Daemen College, Amherst, New York

Priscilla L. Sagar, EdD, RN
Assistant Professor, Division of Nursing, Mount Saint Mary College, Newburgh, New York

Linda J. Scheetz, EdD, RN, CS, CEN
Professor and Chair, Division of Nursing, Mount Saint Mary College, Newburgh, New York

Linda S. Smith, DSN, RN
Assistant Professor, School of Nursing, Oregon Health Sciences University, Klamath Falls, Oregon

Vicki L. Smith, MS, RN
Instructor, College of Nursing, Niagara University, Niagara, New York

Elizabeth N. Stokes, EdD, RN
Associate Professor, and Director, Master of Science in Nursing Program, Department of Nursing, Arkansas State University, Jonesboro, Arkansas

Anita L. Throwe, MS, RN, CS
Associate Professor, Medical University of South Carolina, College of Nursing Satellite Program at Francis Marion University, Florence, South Carolina

Geraldine Valencia-Go, PhD, RN, CS
Associate Professor, and Director, GAINS Project, School of Nursing, College of New Rochelle, New Rochelle, New York

Ann H. Venuto, MS, RN
Instructor, College of Nursing, Niagara University, Niagara, New York

Sandra B. Weatherford, MSN, RN, FNP, CEN
Instructor, Medical University of South Carolina, College of Nursing Satellite Program at Francis Marion University, Florence, South Carolina

PREFACE

When I first proposed this book to the publisher, I was asked what would make it stand apart from all the other nursing education books on the market. The answer to that question and my goal in producing this book was simple—to develop a "user friendly" resource for nursing faculty as they move along their career paths, especially in those early years. As chairperson of a nursing division, I am acutely aware of the need for new faculty to get started on the "right" path early—the tenure track clock ticks quickly. From landing that first position in academe to preparing for tenure review, this book addresses frequently asked questions posed by faculty in their "early" years. The book concludes with several case studies of particularly challenging situations.

This book is not intended to be a comprehensive or prescriptive text to guide nursing faculty. Rather, it is intended to be a resource to support faculty in the early years of their career—a resource that offers the wisdom and experience of faculty who have succeeded in the sometimes mysterious world of academe. I have been searching for many years for a book like this to share with new faculty.

I was convinced of the need for this book, and at the same time, curious to see what interest there would be among my nurse faculty colleagues. I can only say that I was pleasantly amazed at the response to my call for authors. So many talented, experienced nurse faculty responded that it was a challenge to select those few who would contribute. Several of these talented faculty proposed interesting ideas for chapters that I had not thought of when I first conceived the idea for this book. Their ingenuity and insights have made this book far better than what I had envisioned. Faculty who contributed to this book are a diverse group representing public and private schools, secular and nonsecular schools, community colleges, small liberal arts schools, comprehensive universities, and academic health science centers. Their collective wisdom and advice should benefit us all.

I offer this book to you, the committed community of nursing faculty, who never have enough hours to do all those things you believe are important, but who still manage to educate the finest cadre of nurses in the world. I hope this book provides some quick answers to those pesky questions that keep us awake at night.

Linda J. Scheetz, EdD, RN, CS, CEN

Acknowledgments

No one undertakes the writing of a book without the help and support of others. I owe a particular debt of gratitude to Linda Belfus, President of Hanley & Belfus, for believing in me and having the courage to venture away from her company's highly successful series of medical Secrets books to allow me to write a Secrets book about nursing education. A special thanks to Ernest Mills, III, for his thoughtful critique and suggestions related to the chapter on Legal and Ethical Issues. I am also grateful to my faculty colleagues at Mount Saint Mary College for their willingness to review various drafts of the book and their patience with me when I was totally engrossed in editing this book. Last, but certainly far from least, is my gratitude to the chapter authors for their tireless effort, enthusiasm, and wisdom in writing their manuscripts and meeting my deadlines.

I. Higher Education and the Faculty Role

1. LANDING THAT FACULTY POSITION: A VIEW FROM BOTH SIDES

Linda S. Smith, DSN, RN

VIEW FROM THE PERSPECTIVE OF A NURSING FACULTY POSITION SEEKER

1. What do I need to decide before I begin my job search?

The first decision to make is, "Should I seek a new position?" The second determination is really a series of questions and decisions focusing on:

- when to search
- what type of institution—large/small, research/teaching, union/nonunion, public/private, andragogical/pedagogical, traditional/innovative
- location—local/regional/national/international, urban/rural
- living environment (e.g., culture, transportation/access, sports, housing, leisure opportunities)
- who (who will be affected and how)

Spend careful time with these decisions; consult family, friends, advisors, and trusted colleagues. Place the results of your decisions on a rating scale of importance (for example, a 1 to 5 Likert, with 5 being extremely important, 1 being of minimal concern). This prioritization scale will serve well during the entire search process, especially when compromises are needed. The last decision, of course, comes much later in the hunting process, "Should I accept this offer?"

To answer many of these questions, personal and professional philosophies need to be considered and documented. Answers to, "How will my philosophical views blend with those of the program and institution?" will be possible only when your beliefs are clearly stated in writing.

2. What do I need to prepare?

The following materials should be prepared prior to beginning your search:

- Professional teaching and research philosophies (written)
- Current, perfectly produced curriculum vitae (CV, vita)
- Evidence of teaching abilities (i.e., student evaluations, videotape of actual class, administrative reports, syllabi)
- Evidence of scholarly work (a dissertation abstract, published articles and books, research summaries—past and current)
- References (at least one reference each that will speak to research potential, teaching, teamwork); a dissertation or thesis advisor is an excellent choice. Always tell potential referees of your plans and seek permission for the inclusion of their names as job references.

For the purpose of easily retrieved transcripts and error-free applications, prepare a chart of all post-high-school educational facilities attended. For each school, include current transcript cost, contact (address, phone, fax), requirements (e.g., a signed, dated request letter), turnaround times, dates of attendance and graduation, and number of credits earned. Though many search committees will not need transcripts with an initial application (but they may ask for noncertified photocopies), these documents will be needed for license endorsement and degree verification once a position has been secured. Create a similar list for all nursing licensure and certification credentials. *Hint: A great many details can be verified by accessing Board of Nursing and university web pages.*

The application packet should include a cover letter (indicating how you learned of the position, your qualifications for the position), clearly identified ways to reach you, and your interest in the stated position. Then, in order, address exactly those qualifications noted in the job ad. References may be solicited from each referee or from a university-based credential file. Either way, send names, addresses, phone numbers, and email locations with the application packet. Many (maybe most) search committees contact referees by phone, even when letters are available.

Mail application packets using a tracking system such as UPS or certified mail. Thus, receipt of these important materials is verifiable. Expect to receive an affirmative action card a week or two after your packet has been received. Complete and return this card immediately (yes, it is voluntary).

3. Where do I look for nursing faculty position openings?

Many potential employers of nursing faculty advertise available positions in professional publications, including The Journal of Nursing Scholarship, AJN, and American Nurse. The Chronicle of Higher Education offers one of the most extensive, searchable databases for faculty job seekers. Many universities have placed The Chronicle on their permanent and constant list for publishing administrative and faculty positions. Best of all, free web access is available even to nonsubscribers (subscribers can access ads before they are published) with easy search and retrieval mechanisms. The Chronicle offers free weekly email notification of available nursing-related positions. These job ads almost always include links to university web sites, allowing potential candidates to obtain additional information while saving time. Useful articles are also displayed. The web site address is <www.chronicle.com>; click 'jobs' key word 'nursing' (with limit capabilities by region and country). A list of all nursing-related positions with links to actual job postings will be displayed.

In addition to The Chronicle's web site, try the Academic Position Network at <www.apnjobs.com/apn.html>. Sort by country, field of interest (nursing), position type (faculty, administration), and institution type (research, vo-tech, etc.). Black Issues in Higher Education can be accessed at <www.blackissues.com>. Click job announcements/position announcements and search (past or current issues). Subscriber status is required for job postings; however, free access to current news and articles is available. Another general job search site is <www.americasemployers.com/advertised/>, and click on academic positions. This site offers help with improving job search skills. <Monster.com> can be used if identifying nursing as a search term and faculty as sub-search. Additionally, <Monster.com> has general resources such as resume and cover-letter dos and don'ts and sample resignation letters.

One web site specific to nursing, which at the time of this writing is promised but not yet available, is <www.nursingsociety.org>; click on "careers" then "job postings" for current ads. The American Association of Colleges of Nursing job search database is only a click away at <www.aacn.nche.edu>. Follow the links to careers/jobs.

4. Where will I get free job hunting advice and help?

Besides the web sites mentioned, one favorite, <www.rileyguide.com>, has multiple links that answer almost any job search question, including interviewer expectations and the 10 most frequently asked interview questions (www.americasemployers.com/faiq.htm). Another easy and valuable web site is <www.jobweb.org/catapult/jsguides.htm>.

Universities often offer graduates free or low-cost career counseling, campus credential services, as well as resume and interview critiques. An additional free help source includes colleague and mentor input. After accessing helpful job skill web sites, create a list of possible interview questions and have a colleague "interview" you on videotape. This colleague or mentor could also critique your CV.

5. How will I be interviewed?

Candidates are interviewed by telephone conference calls, at regional and national meetings, and during on-site visits. Candidates are most often asked to explain past, present, and future research and teaching interests. The tried and true "Why here; why now?" demands clear, positive, professional, yet brief answers. Expect to answer questions about fundability of your research plans as well as current and future publishing activities (refereed, research journal). Due to budget constraints and careful considerations for time and resource expense, telephone interviews by candidate-seeking individuals and groups are almost always precursors to on-site visits.

6. Should I prepare a presentation?

Yes. If you are invited for an on-site interview, a presentation is almost always expected. Presentation requirements vary, however, and may include demonstrations before an actual class, a description of a teaching technique, or a formal research presentation. *Hint: Be prepared for additional speaking opportunities.* For example, during initial interviews, a topic may surface which becomes a requested presentation subject. Have all equipment in perfect working order. Overhead transparencies are not the best tools to use; think about creating and polishing a computer presentation, using software such as PowerPoint®. During the presentation candidates are evaluated for speaking/teaching abilities, enthusiasm, and ability to answer unexpected questions. Be prepared with handouts. If the school offers to make these for you, be sure they have them at least one week in advance (mail handouts, don't fax them).

7. What can I expect from the on-site visit and how do I prepare?

Expect the unexpected and bring everything you will need. Prepare for on-site visits by learning everything possible about the institution. Collect all web and print sources and compile these sources into a categorized loose-leaf notebook. Categories should include required and recommended nursing courses (circle the courses you would teach or co-teach), faculty members with research histories, program and university sections with philosophies (jot notes on how these blend with yours), accreditation histories, stakeholders, and community/environment. Tabs facilitate easy retrieval. Identify how your strengths would enhance current faculty expertise and program outcomes. The first section in this "school notebook" should be "correspondence" and contain all important documents regarding the visit. Create a second "personal" folder with these categories: CV/personal (include CV, a sample introduction, news announcements, teaching and research philosophies), research (abstracts, proposals), samples of scholarly work (published articles), copies of transcripts and references, and evidence of teaching effectiveness. If your presentation is on PowerPoint®, bring an extra disk copy and copies of any handouts. Your list of questions to ask should also be kept close at hand. Keep these two folders throughout your visit.

Beware of illegal questions. Questions that delve into marital status, ethnicity, age, family planning, sexual orientation, disability, spiritual commitments, etcetera, are illegal. Answer such questions by asking, "How does . . . relate to specific job duties as a nursing faculty member?"

Expect to ask as well as answer questions. Below is a list of possible questions to ask during telephone and on-site interviews:*

- Average weekly faculty work load
- Faculty development mechanisms and monies
- Faculty turnover
- Faculty/student ratio (classroom and clinical)
- How long has coordinator/chair been at her/his job?
- Laboratory—how run and equipped
- Mileage reimbursement for off-campus responsibilities
- NCLEX-RN pass rate
- New faculty orientation
- NLNAC or CCNE accreditation status (number of years accredited and status)
- Number of full-time and part-time faculty
- Office, computer, and library support for faculty
- On-site visit specifics
- Relocation assistance
- Salary and benefits (how much does school contribute)
- Sales tax, state tax
- School/department of nursing budget and chain of authority
- Secretarial support
- Status of the school of nursing within the community and the university
- Student admission and progression processes
- Theoretical framework of the curriculum
- Rank (anticipated range)
- Tenure requirements
- Tuition discount/waiver for self/family
- Type of contract
- Special features

  * ©Smith-Miller Financial Planning, Inc., Klamath Falls, Oregon, 1998. Used with permission. All
     rights reserved.

8. When is it appropriate to discuss issues of salary and rank?

Though a critically important concern for candidates, salary is often not formally mentioned until after the institution has presented its offer. One of the last items on most site visit agendas is a final meeting with the unit administrator. After seeking permission ("Is it premature for me to inquire about potential rank and salary?"), these subjects may be tactfully broached.

9. What are important "dos" for me as a prospective faculty member?

- Create a personal profile that is valued by potential employers, e.g., certification, doctoral preparation, research trajectory, funding history. For example, a short-term interim teaching position may be the best way to establish yourself as a competent educator
- Prepare well for all interviews; have everything you need close and easily retrievable
- Stay flexible, positive, relaxed, and genuine
- Express your desire for the position (if it's true)
- Develop one or more contingency plans

- Be patient and demonstrate a willingness to repeat answers over and over
- Ask questions, shake hands, start conversations, demonstrate interest
- Stick close to your goals and objectives; refer often to the original reasons for this job change
- Immediately inform your potential employer of any changes (airline delays, withdrawal of application)
- Write thank you notes to everyone who has helped you
- Remember, even if you do not accept a position, you have left behind an important impression
- Remember that job hunting is enormously time-consuming and stressful. Stay physically fit, get enough rest, and try to have some fun!

10. What should I never do (when seeking a new position)?
- Use your present employer's email account, fax machines, letterhead, postage, phone lines. This is considered theft.
- Burn bridges
- Renege on an acceptance, even if that acceptance was verbal
- Be dishonest in word or deed
- Allow interruptions during telephone interviews (beepers, pets, family)
- Place presentation, contacts, and interview materials in checked bags
- Become publicly intoxicated
- Slander present or former colleagues and employers

11. How can I make the best possible impression?
- Publicly acknowledging and thanking the hard work of the search committee and chair
- Staying flexible, ethical, adaptable, honest
- Dressing in professional-looking, pressed clothes and shoes
- Proofread everything! (don't forget that electronic communication carries important grammar and format requirements)
- Attend to deadlines
- Get plenty of sleep, eat right, and exercise—stay well; look refreshed

VIEW FROM THE PERSPECTIVE OF
THE NURSING FACULTY SEARCH COMMITTEE

12. Who makes up the search committee?
Usually there is one person, chosen by the program administrator, who functions as chair. This position should be filled by a tenured faculty member. The chair will coordinate all committee meetings and activities. The chair also functions as the contact person for all applicants. Search committees may comprise entire programs/departments if the program is very small. Usually, the committee consists of three or more "volunteers" (ten are too many!) from faculty ranks.

13. Before beginning our candidate search, what does our program and search committee need to prepare?
Prepare careful job descriptions, candidate qualifications, and selection criteria papers. All searches need to begin with a specific set of attributes being sought. These items need to be included in the job advertisement, so do this as soon as an opening is evident. The job description needs to include nursing specialization, duties, required licensure/certifica-

tion/degrees, experience, scholarly activities, and work expectations. Of these criteria, committee members must decide between required and desired.[3]

Next, committee members should create pre-written interview guides and questions (examples are available online), question sheets for candidate references, and evaluation sheets for campus presentations. These will be distributed to all interviewers during telephone and campus sessions. Construct sample letters for these purposes: (a) "We have received your application," (b) "We would like to schedule a telephone interview/site visit," or (c) "Thank you but we are not interested".

14. How might we reduce our advertising costs?

First, be discriminating with advertising dollars. Check the history of other searches. What were the primary sources for the best candidates? Which publications reach the greatest number of potential contestants? Rank order the publications and choose locations based on this ranking. In this current tight job market, a great deal of money is being spent on advertising— make those dollars count.

After carefully formulating a plan, use low-cost and even free advertising mechanisms, such as advertising online (see question 3 in the first section of the chapter), sending out email messages (or printed flyers) to internal and external colleagues and departments, and distributing ad sheets during professional conferences. ***Hint:*** *While attending nursing meetings and conferences, network with peers from other universities, sharing your "good" news.*

Online advertising is increasingly being used by search committees. In addition to the web sites already mentioned, <www.dbm.com/jobguide/post.html> describes how to use the Internet to post openings, how to search for the best people, and how to improve search outcomes.

15. What should we build into our search time line?

When putting together a candidate search time line, expect the unexpected and add plenty of adjustment time. It may take a tremendous amount of time to get approvals for advertisements and funding, and receive transcript and reference submissions. Many professional publications need several months or more of lead time for ads, not counting the time it takes to prepare camera-ready copy. Checking references may take up to 2 weeks of telephone tag. Candidates need 2 or more weeks of lead time prior to any campus visit. This lead time is especially important because air fares are usually significantly higher without a 21-day advance purchase. If administrators must have time with candidates, expect difficulties in coordinating calendars.

16. What are important "dos" for our search committee?

Search committees and programs should:
- Consider all candidates as potential colleagues; treat each applicant with care and respect.
- Keep applicants and candidates informed during all phases of the search process
- To save money, reduce the number of on-site visitors to about two or three per position opening.
- Prepare, coordinate, communicate.
- Inform candidates ahead of time for reimbursable expenses; reimburse these costs immediately.
- Maintain all application materials with strict adherence to confidentiality.

17. What should our search committee never do?
- Be dishonest (about workload, research, advising requirements)

- Hide bad news such as NCLEX-RN scores, loss of accreditation
- Contact applicant references or employers without permission
- Divulge candidate status by phone or email (persons on the other end of the phone may falsely identify themselves!)
- Ask illegal questions such as queries regarding pending offers, current position status, spouse employment, etc. (refer to question 7, section 1)
- Advertise and seek candidates for a position that is already filled
- Carry hidden agendas such as advertising for one type of candidate while seeking something very different
- Ask a candidate to prepare a presentation with less than 2 weeks' notice
- Interview two candidates simultaneously
- Publicly discuss personal, confidential candidate details

18. How should our program and committee prepare for site visits?

To best prepare all persons involved in site visits (candidate, search committee, program staff/faculty, institution, administration), begin by deciding who will pay for expenses and how these costs will be reimbursed. Remember, it can be an unfair burden for candidates to carry campus-visit costs (sometimes more than $1,000), even if those expenses are reimbursed later. Provide candidates with date options (they are busy and must juggle multiple responsibilities). Choose these options after attending to the schedules of administration, students, faculty, and staff. Create an agenda and send it to candidates as soon as possible. Be sure to give each applicant clear details regarding his/her presentation, such as who (who will be the audience and how many are expected), *where, when, why,* and *how* (describe any equipment and materials candidates will need to bring). Identify what will be expected during the presentation and question/answer periods.

Construct an agenda that provides for rest periods yet allows the institution and applicant a good view of each other. Candidates will welcome opportunities to visit with benefits personnel, tour campus facilities (library, research, skills lab) and community areas, speak with realtors, meet informally with program colleagues, and talk to students. Search committees will want to see the candidate interact in formal as well as informal settings. Finally, remember to inform candidates of when and how they will be informed of the search outcome.

19. What can our search committee do to save time and money?

To save time, embarrassment, and money, the search committee and chair should keep track of every step of the process by creating a database, available on a network drive, with pre-identified variables and codes. This database will contain details of:
- When application was received, what was missing, when missing items were received
- When the "we've received your application" letter was sent
- Results of the first screening and when the "we're not interested" letters were sent
- When references were checked and with whom
- Date of telephone interview(s) and results
- Date of site visit and results

20. What questions should be asked when checking references?

Questions to referees of potential candidates are often based on issues raised during the candidate credential review and interview. Sometimes, the questions need to be very direct and personal. At other times, questions may be geared toward the structures and political function of the school and university. Three questions commonly asked include:
- What is it really like to work with this person?

- What are this person's strengths?
- What are her or his weaknesses?

Other common questions address areas such as teaching ability, teamwork, scholarship, flexibility, levels of enthusiasm to serve institution/department, ability to problem-solve, independence, demonstrated caring toward colleagues/students, and computer skills and experiences.[6] Of course, search committee members need to be aware that people serving as referees may or may not be truthful.

21. How (and why) can we make the best possible impression on potential candidates?

Programs of nursing need to function as a unified whole. Hiring new members of the "team" carries great responsibility and importance. Choosing the wrong person is expensive and potentially harmful. That is why the search committee needs to understand that a good search is a two-way process of fit. Even if applicants are not chosen or choose not to accept, they will still remember and talk about their experiences for many years. And who knows, these same applicants may be back in a year or two for the next vacancy. Just as with taxes and death, candidate searches are a sure thing!

BIBLIOGRAPHY

1. Cole BR: Applying Total Quality Management Principles to Faculty Selection. Higher Educ 29:59-75, 1995.
2. Gappa JM, MacDermid SM: Work, Family and the Faculty Career. New Pathways: Faculty Career and Employment for the 21st Century Working Paper Series, Inquiry #8. Washington, DC, American Association for Higher Education, 1997.
3. Greene TJ, et al: Conducting a faculty search. ASEE Prism 5:26-31, 1996.
4. Heiberger M, et al: The Academic Job Search Handbook, 2nd ed. Philadelphia, University of Pennsylvania Press, 1996.
5. Murray JP: Hiring the faculty for the next millenium. J Staff Prog Organ Devel 16:5-14, 1998.
6. O'Neill M: Questions to Pose to Candidate References. State University of West Georgia Department of Nursing Search Committee proceedings, unpublished, 1999.
7. Perlman B, McCann LI: Recruiting Good College Faculty: Practical Advice for a Successful Search. Bolton, MA, Anker Publishing Co, 1996.
8. Ryan M, et al: An analysis of faculty recruiting in schools and departments. Journalism Mass Commun Ed 50:4-12, 1996.
9. Savory PA: Making the move from student to teacher: Steps in the faculty search process. IIE Solutions 26:60-63 , 1994.

2. GAINING PERSPECTIVE:
ORGANIZATIONAL STRUCTURE

Mary Lou Rusin, EdD, RN

1. What is the difference between a college and university?

The common purposes of institutions of higher learning include teaching, research, and public service. Though both colleges and universities are considered institutions of higher learning, universities have a broader and more comprehensive focus. Universities typically have reputations in teaching and research, and are corporate bodies empowered to award a wide array of degrees. There are usually graduate and professional schools that offer masters and doctoral degrees, and undergraduate divisions that award baccalaureate degrees. Universities have a strong emphasis on research as part of their mission statement.

Colleges are usually viewed as having a junior status to universities but may also award both undergraduate and graduate degrees. Ordinarily, there is more emphasis on teaching than on research in small colleges, while a large university with multiple graduate programs and research and service components may emphasize teaching, research, and public service.

The organizational structure of colleges and universities also varies. Typically, colleges and universities are organized on a line-staff basis with clearly delineated reporting relationships. Since colleges tend to be smaller, their administrative line structure is also less complex than that of universities. Regardless of size and/or complexity, most college and university organizations include four major administrative areas: academic affairs, business management (including financial and property), student services, and development and external affairs.

2. What is the difference between a college of nursing, school of nursing, nursing division, and nursing department?

All of these titles are designations for the nursing unit within a college or university; the difference in terminology relates to the organizational structure of the parent institution. Departments are the basic organizational building blocks of colleges and universities. The chief nurse administrator may be referred to as a chairperson, dean, or director, depending on the constitution of the parent institution (refer to the table in question 5). In large universities, the nursing unit is often referred to as the nursing division or nursing school or college, whereas at smaller, less complex colleges, the term nursing department describes the nursing unit.

3. How does the nursing program fit in with the rest of the college or university?

To understand the question of "fit," it is important to compare the stated mission and goals of the university or college with those of the nursing program. In fact, this "fit" is an important element to consider in light of the standards set by specialized nursing accreditation bodies such as the National League for Nursing Accrediting Commission (NLNAC) and the Commission on Collegiate on Nursing Education (CCNE). Both accrediting organizations place great emphasis on consistency of the mission and goals of the nursing program and those of the institution as a whole. Nursing programs fit well within institutions that espouse a humanitarian service component as part of their mission.

4. Who is my boss?

Reporting relationships for nursing faculty depend on the administrative organization and complexity of the institution and that within the nursing program. In large schools, faculty may not report directly to the dean or chair, but to an intermediary administrator such as an associate dean or graduate director. Many larger programs of nursing formulate a set of bylaws, which define the reporting lines and channels of communication. Typically the dean or chairperson of the nursing unit is either selected by the president or academic vice president (provost or dean), or is elected by the department members.

The dean or chairperson of the nursing unit has many responsibilities that vary with the size and complexity of the parent institution. Generally, budget formulation, selection and retention of academic staff, interdepartmental relationships, educational development, faculty development, student advisement, college/university committee participation, class scheduling, student records, faculty load, and initiation of curriculum changes are among the basic tasks the chairperson is responsible for. Deans of nursing units within large university settings may also determine faculty promotion and tenure, develop research grants, and provide a liaison between the nursing faculty and central administration of the parent institution.

5. I've heard of presidents; what are deans, provosts, and chancellors? What do they do?

The basic organizational structure of academic institutions and nomenclature for academic administrators varies widely and depends on the objectives, size, and complexity of the college or university, and the individual institution's philosophy of education. The table below depicts the differences in titles based on size of the parent institution.

Titles of Academic Administrators

INSTITUTION TYPE	CHIEF EXECUTIVE OFFICER	CHIEF ACADEMIC OFFICER	NURSING UNIT ADMINISTRATOR
Four-year college	President	Vice President for Academic Affairs or Dean of the Faculty (or College)	Nursing Department Chairperson or Director or Nursing School Dean
University	President or Chancellor	Vice President or Provost	Dean
Multi-university system	Chancellor	Vice Chancellor	Dean

Presidents (or chancellors) are the *chief executive officers* of the college or university, and have many and varied duties. Their specific responsibilities are defined by the university or college bylaws and contracts, and include duties as members of the governing board and of committees of the board. In the role of executive officer of the board, the president or chancellor is responsible for implementing policies, preparing reports on the official status of the institution, and serving as an ex officio member of board committees. The president, as chief executive officer, is expected to provide general supervision of all aspects of the institution. The administrative responsibilities of the chief executive officer include:
- Approving appointments to the faculty and staff
- Recommending certain appointments to the board
- Recommending policies to the board

- Preparing and administering budgets
- Administering academic affairs and use of the physical plant and facilities
- Supervising public relations, community relations, and alumni relations
- Developing long-range planning (academic and physical) of the institution
- Implementation of fund raising
- Representing the university or college at all functions
- Presiding at or conducting public official functions including commencement and convocation
- Conferring degrees

The *chief academic officer* of the college or university is referred to as the vice president for academic affairs, the dean of the faculty, the provost, or the vice chancellor, again depending on the organization of the institution and based on its size and complexity. This administrator typically reports directly to the president and is responsible for the academic policy and direction of the institution. Working directly with the deans (or chairs) of the departments (or colleges, or schools), the chief academic officer develops quality teaching, research, and service programs at undergraduate, graduate, and professional levels. (S)he may also have general responsibility for the library, registration and records, admissions, technology, and academic and student service areas, including athletics.

6. How are colleges and universities governed?

Colleges and universities are governed by a group of individuals known in most institutions as the "board of trustees" (private sector) or the "board of regents" (public sector). Boards serve as a liaison between the world of learning—the university—and the world of social interest in learning, which includes the procurement of economic resources. The responsibility and authority for the institution are lodged in the governing board, which establishes policies under which the college or university is to be governed. Trustees also consult with institutional administrators to set long-range goals and deal with strategic planning, including budgeting and investing of funds.

The composition of the board, including types and number of members, varies with the institution's size and mission. Trustees are selected for membership in various ways, including appointment, ex officio appointment, election by public vote, and election by an existing board (self-perpetuation). Boards may also include members from various institutional constituencies including alumni, faculty, and/or students. Church-related schools may have board representation from select church organizations. The characteristics of the parent institution directly influence the selection process for board members.

Trustees are organized according to established bylaws or some similar governing document. Boards of trustees establish policies under which the institution is to be governed. This is their primary responsibility, albeit in many circumstances the board has nominal input, and may be cursory (pro forma) in nature.

Officers of the board ordinarily include the chairman, the secretary, and the treasurer. Board committees are established to further the work of policy making for the institution. Smaller boards may have only three to four committees. Larger governing boards may have many committees. These committees most typically include an executive committee, a building and properties committee, an investment committee, a budget and finance committee, an educational policy or academic affairs committee, and a fund-raising committee.

7. What is the difference between a public and private college and university?

There are a number of significant differences between public and private colleges and universities. Public institutions receive both operating and capital funds from public monies, while private institutions typically receive tax funds for capital purposes but not for operating purposes. Sources of income for private colleges tend to originate directly from tuition, fees, and private contributions and endowment funds. Private institutions tend to be more "tuition dependent" than their public counterparts, with tuition and fees paying for a substantial portion of the costs of salaries and benefits for employees, educational services, and operation of the physical plant. Tuition rates are determined by the individual private institution and are commonly based on competitive factors and total operating costs of the college or university.

Another difference between public and private institutions is the determination of the composition of the board of trustees. In public colleges and universities, board members are typically elected or appointed. In some states, the citizens of the state elect the members of governing boards. In the private sector, boards are more commonly appointed and tend to be self-perpetuating; that is, members of the current board appoint new members.

In public, tax-supported colleges and universities, state laws or county ordinances determine the tuition and fee schedules. The United States Congress defines tuition and fees for federally sponsored institutions. The tuition and fees charged by public, tax-supported colleges and universities tend to be nominal for undergraduate education, and substantially lower for graduate education than those of independent, private institutions. State-funded public colleges and universities determine tuition based on student residency. Students who reside outside the state are charged higher tuition fees as "nonresidents." Private colleges and universities do not have differential tuition charges based on residency.

8. What is the difference between a secular and nonsecular college and university?

Nonsecular colleges and universities typically are linked to religious denominations and thus have an emphasis on religious belief systems as a focus of their institutional mission and goals. Secular institutions are not associated with any religious order. Since nonsecular institutions tend to have mission and goal statements directly related to religious belief, employees of these colleges and universities must assess their own spiritual value system to determine their individual "fit" within the parent institution. Add this issue to your rating scale of priorities when you are considering academic positions (chapter 1, question 1)!

9. What is the role of committees in a college or university?

Committees may serve to provide direct input from faculty to the central administration and board of trustees. The existence and operation of such faculty committees (also referred to as senates or councils) are highly dependent on the approval of trustees and administration and the organizational climate of the institution. Legally, the board of trustees is charged with the authority to make binding decisions, but in many instances the governing board delegates some authority to faculty committees in recognition of the faculty's competence and concern in academic affairs. Faculty senates may have legislative authority over a narrow range of issues, but their functional authority extends over a broad range of topics.

There are two types of committees in colleges and universities: standing (permanent) and ad hoc. Ad hoc committees are special committees formed to complete a given task. Usually ad hoc committees are disbanded once their charge has been completed.

The faculty senate, which is a standing committee, has three major functions: (1) legislative, (2) advisory, (3) forensic.

Legislative control of the faculty senate is usually in the areas of curriculum and student affairs. The senate has "effective" control in these areas and their decisions are rarely overturned by the governing board. The **advisory function** of the faculty senate is engendered through the committee structure of the college or university. Typical faculty committees on a campus include budget, physical planning, calendar, academic standards, promotion and tenure, admissions, and faculty development. Here, the senate provides opportunities for consultation; the strength of the faculty input into final decision making depends on the relationships among the board, the President and the faculty. Finally, the **forensic function** of the senate provides a forum for an exchange of ideas.

10. What is participatory governance?

Participatory governance refers to the concept of shared decision making that characterizes the administration of colleges and universities. A notable characteristic of colleges and universities is that their stated goals tend to be ill-defined, ambiguous, and inconsistent. Therefore, the governance of higher education is inclined to be partly collegial, partly hierarchical, and has a widespread dispersion of decision-making authority. Instead of being thought of merely as employees, faculty are often looked to for input regarding significant campus issues. Through committee participation, faculty have direct or indirect input into the decision-making process. Of course, the impact of this input relates directly to the political atmosphere and organizational culture on the campus, and the administrative attitudes of the president and the governing board. In the current period of rapid and unrelenting change, faculties must be willing to make decisions and provide necessary input into the decision-making process in a timely manner. For this to happen, college and university administration and governing boards must clarify authority, responsibility, and accountability for decision making on their campuses.

11. Do faculty really have decision-making authority?

As stated earlier, the board of trustees is the legal agency of governance of colleges and universities. When the administrative structure of higher education is compared with other organizations, however, many differences are apparent. Traditionally, decisions regarding academic affairs, including such things as determination of desired competencies for faculty, recruitment and selection of faculty, and tenure and promotion decisions, require faculty input. The competence and concern of the faculty are often recognized and sought after by the administration and governing board. Thus, in many colleges and universities, faculty have significant input into decision making at multiple levels through the collaborative governance model.

BIBLIOGRAPHY

1. American Association of State Colleges and Universities: Facing Change: Building the Faculty of the Future. New York, 1999.
2. Balderston F: Managing Today's University: Strategies for Viability, Change, and Excellence, 2nd ed. San Francisco, Jossey-Bass, 1995.
3. Bannister G, Bacon PA: From competitive to collaborative governance. Trusteeship 7:8-13, 1999.
4. Birnbaum R: Faculty in Governance: The Role of Senates and Joint Committees in Academic Decision Making. San Francisco, Jossey-Bass, 1991.
5. Dejnozka EL, et al: American Educators' Encyclopedia. New York, Greenwood Press, 1991.
6. Fincher C: The Changing Future of Academic Leadership. IHE Perspectives, Athens, GA, Institute of Higher Education, 1998. http://service.uga.edu/ihe
7. Miller MA: Let's not grind the works to a halt. Trusteeship 6:20-24, 1998.
8. Perley JE: Faculty and governing boards: Building bridges. Academe 83:34-37, 1997.
9. Ramo K: Reforming shared governance: Do the arguments hold up? Academe 83:38-43, 1997.
10. Tierney WG (ed): The Responsive University: Restructuring for High Performance. Baltimore, MD, Johns Hopkins University Press, 1998.

3. THE ROLE OF FACULTY WITHIN THE COLLEGE OR UNIVERSITY

Elizabeth N. Stokes, EdD, RN, and Christine M. Henshaw, MN, RN

Generally speaking, the faculty role focuses on teaching, research/scholarship, and service. In academic circles, this is often (in jest!) referred to as the "sacred triad." However, the emphasis on one facet of the role or another varies from college to college, and is primarily determined by the college or university's mission. Roles (and expectations) of faculty in a major research university will be very different from the faculty role and expectations in a community college. Ascertaining the Carnegie classification of a college often provides a clue as to the major role emphasis for faculty. For example, at opposite ends of the continuum, the major faculty emphasis at research universities is research, whereas the major faculty emphasis at some baccalaureate-granting liberal arts college or community college is teaching.

Since the role of faculty often differs significantly between community and senior colleges, this chapter offers perspectives on each. Dr. Elizabeth Stokes, Associate Professor of Nursing at Arkansas State University in Jonesboro, offers a perspective of faculty roles in the senior college/university. Ms. Chris Henshaw, Nursing Instructor at Highline Community College in Des Moines, Washington, offers a perspective of faculty roles in the community college.

SENIOR COLLEGE/UNIVERSITY PERSPECTIVE

1. What is implied by the teaching, research and service missions of the college/university?

Teaching, research, and service are the traditional work of educational institutions offering baccalaureate and graduate degrees. Traditionally, these work areas are viewed as integral parts of the whole. Teachers both impart knowledge and discover knowledge. The results are brought to the classroom and to the public. Service combines teaching and research. Service efforts are often directed toward the general public rather than the student body.

2. How do faculty members relate to the mission of the college/university?

Educational institutions vary in the emphasis placed on each of the three traditional missions. Colleges not offering graduate degrees may view teaching as their primary mission and provide support for the development of teaching. Schools with a historical background in agriculture and technical studies often develop extensive continuing education extension and distance education programs. Many large universities, including academic health science centers, have a strong research emphasis. Faculty responsibilities reflect the emphasis of the university. Promotion, merit, and tenure in a research university may depend on faculty building a strong, funded program of research. In other universities, a wide variety of scholarly activities and/or service endeavors may be considered in evaluating faculty work.

3. What will I be expected to do as a faculty member?

The activities of faculty revolve around teaching and learning. Therefore, teaching will be your primary assignment. Most nursing faculty have both classroom and clinical teaching responsibilities. In conjunction with teaching, you will be expected to participate in meetings relative to your courses and the nursing program.

Committee work (service to the institution) is another faculty activity. Depending on the organizational structure (refer to chapter 2), various levels of committees exist. Commonly, a committee structure is present at the department, school/college, and university levels. Therefore, faculty often serve on committees at each level. A third area of faculty activity—research or other scholarly activities—is also expected.

4. Describe what might be scheduled in a typical work week.
The typical work week consists of classroom and clinical teaching plus meetings. You might have class for 2–4 hours each week. Clinical teaching might involve another 15–20 hours per week. Pre- and/or post-conferences for clinical may be scheduled separately or may be included as part of the clinical day. A clinical course may also include a clinical seminar, usually 1 or 2 hours per week. In addition, you will need to review and evaluate student clinical work on a daily or weekly basis. Notes or observations from clinical supervision need to be recorded promptly. Scheduled course or committee meetings may take 2–4 hours a week.

5. What are some other activities relative to teaching that I need to consider?
Working on future classes typically takes 2–4 hours of preparation for each new class hour. Less time will be needed if the class has been taught previously. If class is already organized, your review in preparation for class may take an hour or more. You will want to peruse the textbook material, scan articles, and review notes. Audiovisual materials should be previewed well before class time. Formulating test questions is another time-consuming activity. More about these activities in the chapter on classroom teaching!

6. What about committee meetings?
Committee meetings often require preparation; therefore check the meeting agenda ahead of time. You may need to read and respond to proposed policies or other materials. If faculty are responsible for preparing reports or formulating polices/materials for consideration, these should be prepared and distributed to other committee members before the meeting.

7. What about scholarly activity?
Nurse faculty are engaged in research or other scholarly activities. In planning such activities, establishing a time line is important. Think about the activities that need to be accomplished. Break them down into manageable tasks. Schedule time (and write on your calendar) to work on research or other projects. Determine when and if large blocks of time are needed. Negotiate with your dean for the time needed. Making time for scholarly activity is often difficult. When research or scholarly activity is not funded or minimally funded, time is a precious commodity. Time for funded research or assigned projects may be inherent within the activity. The realities relative to scholarly activity for many nurse faculty is that much work is accomplished outside a normal work week. The chapter on research and scholarship provides additional insights into this valued activity.

8. I am getting started with a small research project or scholarly activity. What support might be available?
Check university/school policies. In some settings, faculty can request a one-course reduction in workload (for a semester) for a specific scholarly activity or research project. The university might provide funds for the nursing program to employ a temporary replacement faculty member for the term. Funds for beginning projects may be available from the school. The local chapter of Sigma Theta Tau or your state nurses' association may also have some start-up monies. Additionally, universities may have small grant funds. Some universities also have "seed money" for beginning researchers.

9. Who decides what I will teach?

Your teaching assignment will depend on your area(s) of expertise and the needs of the program. A dean or department chair may make the overall assignment. Assignments are also governed by whether the new faculty joins a team of teachers or has total responsibility for a whole course. All teaching may be done in teams or with some team teaching and some total course responsibilities. When teaching in teams, the actual assignment of course content may be made by the course coordinator or the faculty teaching team. Teaching assignments may be made in an autocratic or democratic manner. Sometimes the new teacher gets the leftovers after more experienced faculty have made their choices!

10. How do I get started with teaching?

The most urgent initial work of new nurse faculty (whether novice or experienced) focuses on the teaching assignment. The teaching assignment may include a course, or courses, and clinical teaching. New faculty should begin to gather resources for teaching. The textbook may or may not have been chosen. A desk copy should be provided for your use. Publishers generally provide desk copies of textbooks. Check with the publisher about availability of instructor's guides, test banks, and any media. Ask for any previous syllabi, notes, and handouts. Check for audiovisual resources already available.

11. What do I need to do to get started with clinical teaching?

Arrange a meeting with personnel in the clinical area. Often, a more experienced faculty member will accompany new faculty to the initial meeting. New faculty should have some idea from discussions with other faculty about the level and expectations of students. Discuss the mechanics of making student assignments, providing information to staff, and making the experience beneficial to both students and the nursing unit. Faculty new to an agency should arrange for a tour of the facility and the assigned unit (as appropriate). After a tour, new faculty may wish to explore the assigned unit on their own. An orientation by the nurse manager is often in order. If one is unfamiliar with the clinical agency, parts of the employee orientation program may be useful. Be sure to review policies and procedures of the clinical facility before you begin clinical!

12. What else would be helpful in working with students in a clinical area that is new to me?

Consider working with a staff nurse on the unit for a period of time to become familiar with the personnel and patients. Taking a reduced or regular work assignment may be helpful in increasing your comfort level and establishing credibility. Some nurse faculty find it useful to work as staff nurses on a nursing unit where they work clinically with students.

In the first weeks of a clinical experience, periodic dialogue with the nurse manager and nursing staff will help both faculty and students to have a positive experience. A very important strategy for success is establishing and keeping open the lines of communication. Talk to all the personnel on the unit. The unit secretary, for instance, may have ideas about how to facilitate the work with additional people present.

13. What are the expectations of nurse faculty outside the work setting?

Nursing faculty are often expected to belong to and participate in the activities of professional organizations. Most faculty work with both their professional association and specialty nursing groups. Nursing faculty may work with other groups as well. Lay or community groups profit from nursing participation. Female nurse faculty may join women's business/professional groups. An added benefit here is the mutual support of women and representation of nursing in such groups. Nurses who belong to these groups are often instrumental in obtaining scholarship support for nursing students.

Another area outside the work setting is lay support groups. Nursing faculty originally organized a number of support groups throughout the country. Nurse faculty may advise, lead, or convene support groups. Nurse faculty are ideal for such work because of their expertise and leadership ability. Although nurse faculty may participate in extra work activities as described from a sense of mission or professional interest, the university views this as a part of faculty's service contribution to the profession and community.

14. What about professional competence and the maintenance of skills?

Professional competence is important for nursing faculty. Guidelines from the Joint Commission on Accreditation of Healthcare Organizations include requirements for evidence of monitoring competence of employees. Faculty, individually or as a group, must decide what activities generate competence and identify ways to maintain skills. Working as a staff nurse on a periodic basis is one way to maintain professional competence. Spending time with nurses on units where student clinical supervision is done is another way to maintain competence. Faculty may work out agreements to attend agency in-service programs on new equipment, policies, or procedures. For example, undergraduate faculty in one agency participated in sessions for computerized documentation in order to be competent to assist students in working with the new documentation system.

15. Is professional practice important for nursing faculty?

The issue of professional practice for faculty is laden with controversy. While most nursing faculty would agree that maintaining competence and knowledge of practice issues is best accomplished by faculty practice, the issues revolve around the workload of the faculty member. In reality, the faculty workload triad of teaching, service, and scholarship is demanding and leaves little time for practice outside the faculty role. In institutions where professional practice is calculated as part of the faculty member's workload, the issue of finding time for professional practice is more easily resolved.

The following list of questions related to faculty practice should be considered by nursing faculty. Your personal philosophy or the school's philosophy relative to these questions may impact the "fit" between you and the nursing program.

- Should all faculty be engaged in practice?
- What kind of practice should faculty engage in?
- What sites are available for advanced practice for faculty?
- When do faculty find time for practice?
- Will time for practice be a part of faculty workload?
- What about payment for practice?
- Will payment be a part of the faculty member's salary?
- If time for practice is part of the faculty member's workload, does the money earned from faculty practice belong to the school or to the faculty member?

Schools offering advanced practice nursing programs often have faculty-run clinics that afford faculty and students an arena for practice. In such settings, faculty practice generates revenue for the school and the faculty member. Conflicts may arise between faculty who have the potential for this type of revenue-generating practice and faculty without the potential.

In order to maintain certification for some nursing specialties, a specified amount of practice is required. Depending on the specialty, clinical supervision of students may be counted as part or all of this requirement.

16. If practice is expected, how does this fit with the traditional teaching, research and service missions of the university?

Various models of faculty practice already exist. In some instances, the practice component may be designated as service. Teaching may also take place during practice. A nurse midwife faculty member may be precepting a student during scheduled practice time.

Finding time to practice and negotiating money issues must be resolved. Some nursing programs have been able to work out satisfactory plans for practice and teaching, including financial arrangements. Other schools and faculty may encounter problems when practice is not viewed as part of the teaching, research, or service roles of faculty.

17. What is a joint appointment?

A joint appointment is a job for two institutions at the same time. Usually joint appointments involve a clinical agency and the nursing unit within the college or university. Varying percentages of work (time spent) may be negotiated between the two institutions. Salary is often paid on the basis of the negotiated percentage. One example is a faculty member who works 50% for a hospital research department and 50% for the college/university. Another example is a nurse educator in a public health agency who spends 25% of his/her work time coordinating and facilitating baccalaureate student clinical experiences and the remaining 75% of his/her time in the role of nurse educator for the agency.

18. How does the role of nursing faculty differ from that of faculty in other diciplines?

One difference between nursing faculty and faculty in other disciplines is the typical teaching assignment. In other disciplines, a faculty member may teach four sections of the same course or three sections of one course plus one other course. Nursing faculty rarely teach multiple sections of the same course. Although science faculty may teach laboratory sections of a course, times for these courses are often two to three hours. (Science faculty might teach 9 hours of course lectures plus 4 hours of lab, totaling 13 scheduled hours in a week. In contrast, nursing faculty might teach 4 hours in the classroom and 20 hours in the clinical area in a week.)

Faculty in other disciplines do not teach practicum/clinical in the same way that nursing faculty do. Precepted experiences are heavily used by other disciplines, such as teaching, physical therapy, and radiologic sciences. In these disciplines, students are assigned to school or clinical agency employees who work with students in their respective areas. The preceptor or supervising teacher has more responsibility for both the clinical experience and the evaluation of the student than is typically found in nursing.

Nursing uses a preceptor model for selected experiences at the graduate level. When preceptor models are used, faculty make site visits. Varying degrees of supervision may be done onsite by nurse faculty. Nurse practitioner faculty may spend a day with a student reviewing their ongoing clinical work.

19. There's so much to do, how should I organize my work?

Think about your organizational preferences. Make lists or set up reminder files. Lists can be labeled by days of the week, by weeks, or months. Reminder files may be organized by time (days, weeks, months) and/or by projects. A plan for work or projects may be written on the file folder or attached to the folder.

Develop a good filing system! Notices, minutes, policies, committee work, and correspondence should be organized in files. A secretary may be helpful in setting up your filing system. Filing systems may be set up by subject areas or in alphabetical order. *Hint: Filing articles under X for Xerox is not very helpful!* For teaching, course materials may be organized in notebooks or file folders. A notebook or a file with reference material pertinent to classes or content areas may also be helpful. This writer maintains a teaching resource file organized by subject.

Think about the tasks to be done. What tasks require blocks of time? What tasks can be accomplished in short time periods? Grading a set of essay papers may be done best in a block of time. Phone calls may be made or returned during short periods of time. Reading material for committee minutes can usually be done in short time periods or will withstand interruption. Likewise, short periods of time or interruptions do not usually hamper answering regular electronic mail messages. However, responding to students using electronic bulletin boards or discussion groups requires that the faculty read at least one message and compose a response without interruption.

20. What activities should take priority?

Initially, teaching activities take priority. Classes must be prepared. Tests must be compiled and administered. Grading and other evaluation should be done in a timely manner. Students should have timely information about their performance in order to learn what growth is needed. Although this area may be problematic, faculty should strive to provide appropriate feedback to students during the term. Lack of timely information about performance is a common complaint of students. If you plan a career in the academic arena, you must plan to develop professionally in teaching, scholarship, and professional service. Thinking and planning in all areas from the beginning will foster a successful career.

21. What are some suggestions about pulling all of this (teaching, research, service) together?

The expectations of nursing faculty are often overwhelming. The challenge is to find ways to work smarter, not harder! The demands of teaching, particularly in the clinical area, and committee work "eats" time. Finding ways to combine the responsibilities of teaching with research and/or service is one way that faculty can work smarter. *Hint: Be aware of tenure, promotion, and merit guidelines from day one!* Scholarly work should fit within those guidelines. If acceptable, research related to teaching may be undertaken. Papers or presentations detailing innovative or new teaching approaches are a way of combining expected faculty work. Establishing projects that provide teaching, research and service are an ideal way to combine all expected faculty work. One example is that of a nurse faculty who initiated an extension of a home health program as a clinical learning site for students. The program provided both a teaching site and served the community. Faculty and students in the new program were involved in research about the outcomes of the new program. Collaborative research with other faculty and/or clinical agencies is another example of working smarter.

22. What about working with students on scholarship or research projects?

Working with undergraduate or graduate students is also a way of being involved in scholarly activities or conducting research. This writer and another faculty member conducted a curriculum project with a graduate student. In another instance, a student interested in research wanted additional experience in reading and interpreting research findings. The student, in an independent study course, produced a literature review on lay support groups. *Hint: When working with students, be clear about ownership, authorship, and future use of work.*

23. What rules govern my behavior?

Both official and unofficial rules govern faculty behavior. Official statements are found in various handbooks published by academic units. The university also has a faculty handbook that contains general policies and rules. Examples include policies about sick leave, outside employment, consultation, and the production of creative works. Faculty handbooks usually contain statements about misconduct. Falsifying information, sexual harassment, assaulting other faculty or students, and research misconduct are examples of conduct that may warrant dismissal.

Although teachers are role models, the days of very strict behavior codes are bygone. Faculty are generally expected to represent the school and the profession in public. Unwritten rules about faculty behavior may include attendance at certain meetings and special academic functions. Faculty should dress using good taste. Some campuses are more informal than others. Faculty are usually more formally dressed than students. Many faculty think that presenting a neat, well-dressed image in the classroom is important. Clothes, appearance, and behavior all communicate to others. Nursing faculty should be clear about the messages they deliver nonverbally through their actions and dress.

24. What other sources provide information about faculty behavior and policies?

Additional handbooks for a college/school/department may have more specific information. Examples of information in these handbooks include responsibilities of course faculty/coordinators, retention of student papers, student dress code, and substance abuse policies. Student handbooks for the university and for nursing students contain additional policies. Grievance procedures, for example, are detailed in university student handbooks. A nursing student handbook might include a list of needed equipment, information about advisement, and specific health regulations.

25. How do I become involved in campus life?

New faculty should attend orientation not only to gain information, but also to begin to meet other people on campus. Attend receptions and parties for new faculty. If there is a newcomers group, join and participate in meetings. If you belong to honor organizations such as Phi Kappa Phi, attend at least some of the meetings. In the absence of a faculty women's group, female faculty members should consider joining the faculty wives' club. Attend these activities for at least a year. Such a group provides the opportunity for developing friendships outside of nursing and also gives one a flavor of the campus. Women in these groups understand academia and are wonderful resources about the community. Faculty wives' groups often offer excellent programs and may engage in service projects (conversations with international students or raising scholarship money, for example). A local chapter of the American Association of University Women is another worthwhile group. Talk to the student services group on campus. You may want to sponsor or advise a student group. Conducting educational or informational programs for dormitory residents is another way to be involved in campus life. Volunteer for an event or group on campus. This writer's campus has a faculty choral group and faculty bell-ringer, as well as a tradition of faculty serving a special meal to students on the Tuesday evening before Thanksgiving. If newer faculty are not readily appointed to campus committees, find someone to nominate you for the faculty senate or other college-wide committee.

COMMUNITY COLLEGE PERSPECTIVE

26. What will I be expected to do as a faculty member?

At the community college, the primary mission is teaching. Faculty workload most often is based on contact time with students, that is, direct teaching time. For example, in a quarter system, an instructor might be required to teach three 5-credit courses. Those 15 credits translate to 15 contact hours, or 15 hours per week directly teaching students.

Other duties directly relate to contact with students. Faculty generally are required to maintain a certain number of office hours per week; 5 hours per week is common. Student advising, both for preprogram students and students within the program, is expected. Faculty may also be expected to provide general advising for students from other disciplines or for students without a declared major.

In addition to direct contact with students, you will be expected to prepare for courses, develop syllabi, and design classroom activities. Participation in curriculum development and revision, as well as attention to the integration of your courses with other courses in the department, requires time and collegial interaction. Maintaining relationships with clinical sites will also be part of the role of clinical faculty.

Beyond the nursing department, you will be expected to participate in the work of the college through participation in committees and task forces, such as campus-wide curriculum development, assessment of student outcomes, and shared governance.

27. Is professional practice important for nursing faculty?

Faculty at community colleges generally are not required by contract to maintain professional practice. More and more, however, service to the community and leadership within the discipline are valued components of the faculty role. Maintaining clinical currency is essential for the vitality of the curriculum and enhances credibility of the faculty with students and agency staff. However, you will most likely be expected to maintain clinical practice on your own time.

28. How does the role of nursing faculty differ from that of faculty in other disciplines?

Depending on the structure of the community college, faculty in nursing may be considered vocational, occupational, or technical faculty, rather than transfer or academic faculty. In many instances, that translates into a different calculation of workload. Where academic faculty might be expected to maintain 15 contact hours per week with students, faculty who teach lab courses, including nursing labs and science labs, may be expected to carry 17-21 contact hours per week.

Nursing faculty, because of the sequential and interrelated nature of the curriculum, spend many hours ensuring an integrated approach to learning. Ongoing discussions of curriculum, expectations, and outcomes are essential to preparing students who meet the qualifications necessary to practice safe and competent nursing.

Nursing faculty teaching a clinical section have a built-in impediment to ongoing participation with other faculty, both within the department and across the campus. Clinical faculty who are off-campus, often 2 days per week, must work extra hard to ensure effective communications with others.

29. There's so much to do, how should I organize my work?

This is a good question to consider during the interview. What are the college's priorities? It might be helpful to check the college and department mission statements. At the community college, teaching and learning are the highest priorities. Attention to classroom preparation and evaluation are number one on the priority list. A weekly planning time can help organize your activities for the week, while maintaining a focus beyond today's demands. On a quarter system, time flies as you are teaching this quarter, preparing for next quarter, and planning curriculum for next year! Juggling all these particulars requires skill and practice.

30. What activities take priority?

Although teaching and learning are paramount, other activities require much time and energy. Keep in tune with the department's and the college's current focus. Perhaps college-wide outcomes are the emphasis. Infusing the curriculum with diversity might be key. The college's strategic plan may help identify some of these areas of focus. Although you may want to keep yourself narrowly focused on the classroom, ignoring the direction in which the college or department is heading will not serve your career path well.

31. What will my schedule be like?

There are as many schedule configurations as there are colleges. However, a typical schedule may look something like this:

Day	*Activity*
Monday	6 hours clinical
Tuesday	6 hours clinical
Wednesday	2 hours classroom 2 office hours 2 hours campus meetings
Thursday	2 hours classroom 2 office hours 2 hours department meeting
Friday	2 hours classroom 2 office hours

Mixed in the "unscheduled" time will be grading papers; preparing classroom activities, including exams; evaluating and grading students; meeting with students unable to come during your office hours; coordinating clinical activities with the clinical site; and doing prep work for committee meetings, among a myriad of other activities that tend to eat up any available free time.

Let's be clear, however. Not all that work will necessarily get done during a 40-hour work week. New faculty, particularly, will find they need time outside the work environment to complete their work. Careful planning and preparation can help minimize the work done on your own time. Setting personal priorities is essential to maintaining a healthy approach to the volumes of work that *could* be done and in focusing on the work that *needs* to get done.

32. What rules govern my behavior?

First and foremost, the signed contract between you and the institution guides your behavior. This may speak only to the number of work days per year. If faculty are represented by a union, the negotiated agreement will spell out the working conditions, including workload, salary, sick time, and expectations. Even if you are not a member of the union, this document provides the standards to which you will be held. Tenure guidelines describe the expectations for achieving tenure. These may be spelled out separately from the negotiated agreement. The department may have other written expectations.

In addition to formal, written expectations, each college has its own culture and climate. While much more difficult to unearth, these unwritten expectations may well be what determines your success in the organization. If these expectations are not written into the negotiated agreement, tenured faculty cannot be fired for failing to meet them. However, when faculty members are perceived as not contributing to the direction of the college, their future requests for special consideration, for grant funds, or for support with special projects may not be granted.

33. How do I become involved in campus life?

Faculty involvement in campus activities is essential for maintaining the life of the college, and is also a source of renewal for the faculty member. Find out about committees and activities on campus, pay attention to oral reports at faculty meetings or to written reports in newsletters, and match your skills and interests with the activities you hear about. Inform your department head of your interest in a particular area, and contact the organizer of the committee or activity that interests you. Committed volunteers are always welcome!

34. Who decides what I will teach?

Although faculty are hired for their expertise in a particular area, flexibility is key. In a department with perhaps only three or four faculty members, you may find yourself stretched to the ends of (or beyond!) your comfort level. A good hiring and selection process increases the likelihood that faculty will teach in their content area. Depending on the size of the department, your teaching assignment may be decided by the department head or by the faculty as a whole. As the curriculum changes and develops, your assignment may change as the focus of the curriculum changes. Be clear about your area of expertise and comfort, but recognize that as the needs of the department change, your assignment may change also.

35. What is the role of a faculty union?

The faculty union represents the faculty in negotiations with the administration. In negotiating the working conditions, the union representatives may consider salary, benefits, workload, faculty expectations, administrative responsibilities, and shared governance. The faculty union also represents individual faculty members in disputes and grievances with administration. The union may coordinate activities such as lobbying in the state legislature or meeting with elected officials. Two of the most common unions representing community college faculty are the National Education Association and the American Federation of Teachers.

36. Who is eligible to join a faculty union?

Eligible members are defined in the negotiated agreement. Generally, all full-time faculty, whether tenured or not, are eligible to join. Part-time faculty may be members of the same union as full-time faculty, or may be represented by a separate bargaining unit.

37. What if my school has a faculty union and I don't want to belong?

Check the agreement negotiated between the faculty and administration. Is the college an open shop? If so, you may elect to not join the union. Your work environment still will be negotiated by the union and you will be covered by the negotiated agreement. Some unions have negotiated an "agency fee." This means you do not have to join the union, but still have to pay a portion of the cost to negotiate the contract, which may be any amount up to and including the same amount as union dues. If the college is a closed shop, you will have no choice: you must join the union.

The final question of the chapter, relating to accreditation, was written collaboratively by Dr. Stokes and Ms. Henshaw.

38. What is accreditation and why is it important?

Accreditation is a voluntary process in which schools or programs engage to assess the status of their educational offerings. Earning accreditation is important because it signifies that the school or program has met specific criteria denoting specific standards. Accreditation standards portray what educators and/or practitioners believe constitutes a quality program. Accreditation communicates to both the profession and society that a program or programs strive to meet standards *above* minimum requirements, and works toward continuous improvement of its educational offerings. Nursing faculty collaborate with other appropriate groups (alumni, nursing colleagues, nursing service personnel, students) in an ongoing process of examining all aspects of the nursing programs in order to graduate competent, marketable *nurses.*

College-wide accreditation is accomplished through meeting the standards of one of several regional accrediting organizations approved by the federal Department of Education (DOE). Although voluntary, any school that wishes to receive federal funds, which includes student financial aid, must be accredited. Following preparation of a self-study report by the college, a team from the regional accrediting body visits the college to ensure that what is claimed in the self-study actually occurs at the college. Full approval results in accreditation for 10 years. Failure to meet the standards of the accrediting body may result in partial accreditation for fewer years, with or without additional visits in between.

Program accreditation, also voluntary, is specialized accreditation that examines a specific program, such as nursing, within the context of the college or university. Currently, two organizations accredit schools of nursing: the National League for Nursing Accrediting Commission (NLNAC) and the Commission on Collegiate Nursing Education (CCNE). NLNAC is an affiliate of the National League for Nursing, whereas CCNE is an alliance of accreditors representing the American Association of Colleges of Nursing and other selected nursing organizations. Both organizations are approved as accrediting bodies by the DOE. CCNE accredits baccalaureate and master's degree programs, whereas the NLNAC accredits all nursing programs from practical nurse programs through master's programs.

The accreditation process should be ongoing, with an emphasis on continued improvement. However, approximately 18 months prior to a scheduled site visit, the nursing program engages in an intensive self-study effort, culminating in a self-study report.

In preparation for a site visit, the nursing department prepares the self-study report, which addresses the following areas: mission and governance, faculty, curriculum, students, and policies. In recent years the emphasis on self-study has shifted from process to outcomes. At a designated time, a team of visitors then visits the college, with directed emphasis on the nursing department to ensure congruence between the report and actual practice. Site visits will last 2 or 3 days, depending upon the size and complexity of the nursing program. During the site visit, the visitors will meet with faculty, students, administrators, alumni, and clinical agency representatives. Additionally, they review written documents such as annual reports, meeting minutes, educational affiliation agreements, handbooks, and catalogs, to name a few.

Full accreditation is granted for 8 years by NLNAC. CCNE grants full accreditation for 10 years. New programs receiving initial accreditation have a shorter accreditation period. Shorter periods of accreditation, with or without interim reports, may also be granted by both organizations if the nursing program does not qualify for a full 8- or 10-year accreditation.

While program accreditation is a voluntary process, it is important to the nursing profession and the public in that it assures compliance with standards that are perceived as important for the education of competent nurses. In addition, program accreditation may be important in articulation to higher levels of nursing education. Many baccalaureate completion, master's, and doctoral programs in nursing require graduation from an NLNAC- or CCNE-accredited school. In addition, entry into the armed forces as a registered nurse requires graduation from an accredited school of nursing.

BIBLIOGRAPHY

1. American Association of Colleges of Nursing: CCNE Accreditation: http://www.aacn.nche.edu/accreditation/index.htm
2. Billings DM, Halstead JA: Teaching Nursing: A Guide for Faculty. Philadelphia, WB Saunders, 1998.
3. Brown HB: Mentoring new faculty. Nurs Ed 24:48-52,1999.
4. Cahill H: What should nurse teachers be doing? A preliminary study. J Adv Nurs 26:146-153, 1996.
5. Macnee CL: Integrating teaching, research, and practice in a nurse-managed clinic: A nonrecursive model. Nurs Educ 24:25-28,1999.
6. Morin KH, Ashton KC: A replication study of experienced graduate nurse faculty orientation offerings and needs. J Nurs Educ 37:295-301, 1998.
7. National League for Nursing Accrediting Commission: Mission: http://www.accrediting-comm-nlnac.org
8. Sherwen, LN: When the mission is teaching: Does nursing faculty practice fit? J Prof Nurs 14: 137-143, 1998.

II. The Sacred Triad:
Teaching, Research, and Service

4. CLASSROOM TEACHING

Sister Leona DeBoer, PhD, RN

1. What is classroom teaching?

A silly question? No, since in our discipline there are such things as clinical teaching, lab teaching, and using the latest technology for distance teaching/learning. Classroom teaching is what goes on in that more formal assembly of students in a room, usually equipped with tables and chairs or student desks, perhaps a blackboard, audiovisual projection equipment and, of course, a teacher.

2. What about the room itself ?

Listen to the wisdom of Florence Nightingale regarding the importance of environment: light, air, temperature, and cleanliness. Attend to these basics and attempt to create a comfortable environment that will be conducive to the teaching-learning process. Students sitting in a dingy, stuffy, cold (or too hot) room will have a hard time focusing on the work at hand. Open the windows, adjust the thermostat, have maintenance replace burned-out light bulbs, have housekeeping dust and sweep once in awhile. It *will* make a difference.

3. What about the furniture?

A table or desk for the teacher should be in the room (you will need a place to spread out course materials you intend to use in the class). Some faculty like to use a lectern. That's OK so long as you do not use it to lean on the whole time! (More on this later.)

Check out the seats students will use. They need something to lean on, too—a table, a writing surface attached to a "student desk." Movable seats are best so that you can rearrange them for small group work and discussion. Obviously, if you have a large class and are assigned to a lecture hall with fixed seating, you will not have this option. Check out size of the seats. Short students' feet may not reach the floor or large students (men, especially) may have a hard time fitting into the seats. If such cases arise, try to influence the facilities/plant manager to make changes. And, of course, report broken furniture to the maintenance department. A degree of seating comfort will enhance the teaching-learning process.

4. Will I need to make arrangements for audiovisual (AV) equipment for my class?

Some classrooms are permanently equipped with basic AV equipment, such as overhead projectors, screens, VCRs, and the like. Many classrooms have become sophisticated with computer-linked multimedia technology. You need to check your classroom ahead of time. Ask yourself these questions: What's available? How do I access it? Do I need orientation/training to use the equipment?

The key here is *plan ahead*. There is nothing worse than to have an entire class go down the tubes due to lack of equipment or equipment that does not work properly. Arrive early to set up and test the equipment before class. Have on hand the phone number of the AV/technology support office in case you need help.

Oh! And don't forget to bring a supply of chalk if you like to use the blackboard, the original visual aid.

5. Now that I have the environment and equipment considered, what about me, the teacher?

First, the *most important* element in classroom teaching is the teacher! Think about it. Without the teacher, you don't need the classroom. The learning can occur elsewhere, anywhere. Here is something to think about:

The mediocre teacher tells
The good teacher explains
The superior teacher demonstrates
The great teacher inspires

(anonymous)

So, let's set about helping you to become that great teacher.

6. My course will be taught through mostly classroom teaching. Where do I start?

A well-developed course syllabus is the essential starting point. It is the blueprint for the course.

7. What should be included in the course syllabus?

The course syllabus, in a sense, is the "teaching-learning contract" with the students. Included in the syllabus should be:

- The course description (verbatim from the college catalog, including credits and pre-requisites)
- The course objectives (or student outcomes, i.e., what will the students know or be able to do by the end of the course?). Make them measurable.
- The required and/or optional textbooks if you choose to have them
- The course calendar (more on this later)
- The unit outline (break the course description into its component topics and make these the units)
- The unit objectives (or student outcomes, i.e., what will the students know or be able-to do by the end of each unit?). Again, they have to be measurable.
- Grading standards (what constitutes an A, a B+, a B, etc.)
- Evaluation methods (what means will you use to measure the students' achievement of the course/unit objectives? exams? assignments? —more on this later)
- An attendance policy if you or your institution require one

8. Do I need a textbook?

Most undergraduate courses incorporate the use of a textbook. Readings from a textbook should be assigned to reinforce and/or to supplement class content. Readings from the text should *not* be a verbatim repetition of what goes on in class. If students can learn all they need to know by reading the text, why is a teacher needed?

Graduate courses, depending on their nature, tend to require a more eclectic approach and/or self-directed student searches for pertinent literature.

9. How do I select a textbook?

Selection of a textbook can be fun. Make friends with the representatives of publishing companies. Let them know what your course is about and they will recommend books published by their respective companies. Many reps visit the schools. Get on their mailing lists. Review copies of texts are easy to obtain through the reps.

Once you have conceptualized the course (developed the course outline/syllabus), review several texts that seem congruent with the course content. Look for reviews written by other faculty; are they favorable? Do the text authors seem reputable/knowledgeable? Are there supplementary materials such as an instructor's manual, transparencies, student workbooks, a test bank? Check the reading level and general appearance, such as size of type and layout. Are graphs, diagrams, and other visuals clear? Are the chapters clearly organized with titles, subtitles, summaries? Is there a good bibliography? Finally, be aware of cost, especially if you think multiple texts are needed for a course. You may want to select a primary *required* text and suggest *optional* texts that students can purchase or have access to in the library.

Having selected the text(s), notify your campus book store in a timely manner so the text(s) can be on hand by the time the course begins.

10.   What about a reading list?

Reading assignments can be listed in a freestanding companion document to your syllabus or you can include them within each unit. How you do this depends on the level and nature of the course. An introductory course may depend primarily on textbook readings. If this is the case, cite the textbook reading assignment in the syllabus within the respective course unit. For an upper level course your expectation may be that students synthesize information from a broader array of resources. In this case the suggested readings can be organized by course units but listed on the companion document. In either case, *be selective.* A short list (3-5) of really pertinent readings that will supplement or reinforce class presentations is best. Long lists of out-of-class readings will overwhelm students to the point that they may do *no* outside reading. Update your reading list *every year*. Also, read the article, report, or book before you assign it. Titles can be misleading.

11.   How do I avoid teaching the whole course on the first day? That is, how do I pace myself?

A course calendar is the first step in pacing yourself. The first time you teach a course, the time-line is a guess, an approximation. Adjustments can and should be made as you go along, and certainly as you plan for the next time you teach the course. Some content just takes more or less time than you originally estimated.

Generate a course calendar by simply listing the dates that the class is scheduled to meet. Do not forget to cross out holidays and school break periods. Next, if you plan to administer exams during part or all of a class period (mid-term, finals, or others), write them in on the respective date(s). Now get your course syllabus and estimate how much time (how many class periods) you will need to cover each unit. Write the unit number and title next to the date(s). Remember, the first time around this is a guess but it should be a reasonable one.

When you distribute the course calendar to the students on the first day of class, be sure to tell them (or write it on the calendar itself) that this is an approximation with regard to the content. Some flexibility ("wiggle room") will be needed. A word of caution: try not to change scheduled exam dates; change only the class content if needed. You do not want the exams to get bunched up.

Use the calendar, the syllabus, and the instructor's manual to plan what you will be teaching on a given date. As you develop this lesson plan (objectives, content, teaching/learning methods), you will find yourself setting priorities about the content for that class. Some things will be "must-do-in-class" that day. Other things can be delegated to ungraded out-of-class assignments (reading, learning exercises, supplementary computer-assisted instruction), and yes, *homework*! For every hour a student spends in class, he or she should expect to spend 2 hours on homework. Clearly inform students of this rule-of-thumb expectation *early* in the course, preferably on the first day.

12.   How much time should I allow to prepare for class?

Several variables impact preparation time: Is this the first time you are teaching the course? How familiar are you with the content? Is this development of a totally new course? Are you teaching a course developed by someone else and for which a syllabus already exists? Is the content related to rapidly changing phenomena?

While answers to these questions may slightly alter the time needed for class preparation, an absolute "must" in all situations is a review of *current* literature (texts, periodicals, research journals) on the class topic, even if you think you are well-versed on the topic. This takes time. Another "there is nothing worse" scenario is to have a student point out that content you are presenting is outdated!

You will need to decide on the teaching/learning methods for the class. If you are preparing a lecture, write out your presentation, even if only in outline form, with enough detail to help you elaborate as you go along. This takes time. If you are planning a small group discussion, prepare the questions, topics, or guidelines for the discussion. This takes time. If you plan to use commercially prepared videos, slides, or transparencies in class, you must preview them ahead of time to ensure they fit with the content. This takes time. If you plan to generate your own transparencies or other audiovisual aids, or if you plan to incorporate presentation software (e.g., PowerPoint7) in your class, this takes time.

And so, the original question does not have a simple answer. You need to "trial run" your preparation until you have some sense of timing. But one thing is for sure, you *do have to prepare*! Students are quick to sense a lack of preparation, usually manifested by disorganization of the lesson, or worse, by outdated content.

13.   How do I get students to prepare for my classes?

Your class presentations, regardless of the teaching methods you use, will be more productive if the students have *also* prepared for them. The most obvious way is to have the students read certain materials (e.g., a related chapter in the text) *before* coming to the class. But guess what! They don't do it!

Some faculty have resolved this problem by having the students (alone or in groups) do, as homework, a short case study related to the upcoming class topic. To answer the questions posed in the study, the students will have to do some reading.

14.   What teaching methods can be used in the classroom?

As many as you can imagine! Lecture, demonstration, questions and answers, role playing, group discussion, debates, and case studies, to name a few. Keep in mind some guiding principles:

- Variety of methods is good. There are diverse ways of learning.
- Use multiple sensory inputs. Some people need a lot of visual prompts; others are auditory dependent.
- Encourage *active* learning. Questions and answers, discussion, writing one-minute papers, e.g., "the most important things I learned in class today were…"
- Have students give examples for the key points of the lesson. "Passive learning" just isn't learning!
- Have high expectations. Continually refer students to the course and unit objectives (outcomes) and help them focus on meeting them. Make the connection between the class content and the objectives.

- Interact with students. Get "up close and personal" by calling them by name, supporting their contributions, gently correcting errors, and moving out among the students, if possible.
- Use a lot of examples, analogies, and images to demonstrate concepts and principles, and to connect new knowledge to students' past experiences and learning. It helps to know how your course relates to the overall curriculum of a program or how your course builds on prerequisite courses.
- Give feedback. Use exams, assignments, and one-minute papers as learning experiences.
- Praise achievement.
- Clarify areas where common errors were made. Guide students to use the feedback to enhance their learning.
- Foster critical thinking. Use learning activities that require students to compare and contrast, to analyze, to synthesize, to apply to new situations, to interpret, to infer, to predict. Nursing case studies are great for this! (Turn to the chapter "Critical Thinking" for more on this topic).

15. What about the lecture method? In this era of "hands on" technology, isn't the lecture method passe?

No! If done well, lecture can be a very effective means of instruction. But let us first define what is *not* meant by "lecture." Academic lecturing should not, in my opinion, consist of reading your notes to a class. A good lecture should incorporate a variety of things to make it dynamic, interesting, and engaging.

- First, be well organized. You do need notes or an outline, but be well-versed enough with the material so that you are not tied to the lectern. *Don't read your notes the whole time.*
- Project the key parts of the outline using a transparency and overhead projector (or presentation software). You can also use that old standby of chalk and blackboard! This will help the students follow your presentation.
- Pace yourself. Present a concept or a principle and then give examples or ask questions to elaborate. Examples from your own experience are attention-getters. Get students to offer examples from their experience. "What if" questions are great to either underscore a point or to demonstrate a counterpoint. Then, go back to your notes to pick up the next section.
- If something is particularly important, say so. Tell students to highlight or somehow mark this "important" in their notes.
- Make use of pauses and repetitions. When you want students to record important points or definitions, go slowly for emphasis. (This is one time you can read your notes verbatim.) Pause to allow them to write. Repeat phrase by phrase, two or three times. When done, scan faces to see if another repetition is needed.
- Use other means of reinforcement, too. Videos can illustrate process and application; however, assign long videos (those longer than 15-20 minutes) for homework rather than using class time. Use the overhead, blackboard, or other visuals for diagrams, illustrations, drawings, and key words.
- Move out among the students, if possible. Leave the lectern frequently, and above all, do not sit at the teacher's desk! Make eye contact. Use gestures and body language appropriately. Be aware of your voice volume and pitch. Be aware of your appearance. It projects an image. Relax and project confidence and enjoyment in what you are doing. It is appropriate to interject a little humor once in awhile, too.
- Leave time at the end of the lecture (or at intervals during it) for questions. Give students time to think and formulate questions. It may help to get them started if you ask

a question or two first. If there is no response give a prompt or rephrase the question. When the students' questions start you can:
- answer them directly
- involve the class in answering them by asking what they think
- acknowledge that you don't know the answer (be honest and nondefensive!) and say "let's look that up and discuss it further in our next class." (Don't forget to do it!)

16. Should I give students copies of my lecture notes?

There are pros and cons to this. If you are well organized and follow a clearly developed syllabus (outline and learning objectives), it is not necessary to distribute your personal lecture notes. Besides, if they are somewhat cryptic with your own shorthand, rubrics, and key phrases that you use to prompt your verbal elaboration, the notes will not be meaningful to students. A good alternative to distributing your notes is the projection of an outline, key words or concepts, diagrams, etc., with the use of transparencies, presentation software, or a blackboard. Some print handouts that replicate your projected material work well, too. But do not drown the students with paper handouts! It is okay to expect them to take notes during a class. (There will also be times when they are writing furiously when you will need to tell them to put down their pens/pencils and listen!)

17. Should I allow students to tape record my lectures?

This depends on how comfortable you are. If you are well-prepared, organized, and confident, why not? Recording the lecture for review and study would greatly help those auditory learners, too. If the student has declared a disability, recording your lecture may be a reasonable accommodation under the Americans for Disabilities Act (turn to the chapter "Students with Special Needs" for a discussion of disabled students). It is a mark of courtesy for the student to request your permission ahead of time, though. Let students know your ground rules for this practice on the first day of class.

18. What other teaching strategies are effective?

While lecture, well executed, can engage students in active learning, several other teaching methods do that even better. Class discussion, role playing, debates, small group problem-solving, simulations, and case studies are effective teaching/learning strategies. The choice depends to some extent on the nature of the course content. Other factors may simply include the physical structure of the classroom itself (e.g., movable seats for small group work). These methods require just as much (if not more) preparation as the lecture method. While these methods have flexibility, they still require a degree of organization and structure to guide students through the exercise in such a way that the learning objectives are achieved. There are more "straying" opportunities with these methods and you need redirection and contingency plans. Increasing student activity in the learning process does not mean that you, the teacher, will be less active!

A good overview of some of the methods is presented in Schoenfeld and Magnan.[6] These authors reference additional resources as well.

19. How do I encourage students to participate in class, regardless of the teaching method?

Some methods, such as role playing and debating, have built into them student participation. Others, such as problem-solving and case studies, require an end-product, such as a report or a conclusion. Students cannot avoid participation with these methods!

Class or group discussion, and even the lecture method, require active student involvement. Try these interactive strategies to engage the students:
- Use questions and answers to summarize content.

- Pose "what if" questions to elicit points and counterpoints, especially when there are pros and cons.
- Get students to give examples from their own experience for a particular concept or principle. Their clinical work is a good source of examples, as might be family life or dorm life. You can "prime" this by first offering an example from your own lived experience.
- Solicit opinions and interpretations.
- Beyond interactive strategies you need to use some personal communication skills:
  - Establish good rapport with the students.
  - Call students by name and acknowledge their contribution.
  - Scan their faces and establish eye contact. Do not forget those seated in the back of the room!
  - Do not be daunted by silence. You need to wait long enough for students to collect their thoughts. Sometimes rephrasing the question is needed.
  - Your outgoing, assertive students will usually get the ball rolling, but do not let them dominate. Often eye contact and an encouraging nod will get a reticent student to respond.
  - If all else fails, call on someone by name to respond to your question, or to offer an opinion, i.e., " . . . and what do you think about the matter, Joe?"

20. How should I respond if a student gives incorrect information during class?

Incorrect information has to be corrected *gently*. You don't want to squelch student initiative and dialogue or belittle the student. Try bringing the rest of the class into the correction: "That's an interesting idea, Joe . . . I wonder what the rest of the class thinks about Joe's idea?" Usually the correct information comes out and you can affirm it by something like, "Yes, in this situation that's probably a better idea. Joe, do you see the difference?"

21. What should I do if a few students monopolize the class participation?

If they do not get the message by your deliberate attempts to involve reticent students, you may have to quietly take aside the dominant students after class and simply ask them to hold back a little (after you thank them for their interest). Do not embarrass them by addressing the problem in front of the other students. Talk with them about helping you support the learning environment with sensitivity and respect for the participation of all students.

22. What about the really disruptive student? How do I handle this situation?

As faculty, you do have to maintain an environment conducive to learning. This implies exercising a certain amount of discipline. If the strategy delineated in question 21 does not work, you may need to enlist the help of student personnel (dean of students, counselors). Arrange a meeting with the student, a counselor, and yourself to address the problem. Keep the discussion focused on the behaviors that disrupt the learning environment. Engage the counselor in helping the student change the disruptive behaviors. If the disruptive behavior got to this point, you may be dealing with a student who needs psychological help. Let the counselor take it from there and make the appropriate referrals.

23. How do I know if my students are learning what I want them to learn?

Assessment of student learning is directly related to the course objectives (or outcomes). So, go back to your syllabus. What did you say at the beginning about what students will know or be able to do when they finish a particular unit or the course? Then, creatively design some ways that the students can demonstrate what they know or what they can do. Of course, the traditional means of assessing student learning are:

- written exams
- formal papers
- projects
- short, focused assignments
- competency (skill performance) exams

Don't forget the homework assignments and one-minute papers (see question 14 above). While you may not assign a formal grade to these, they will give you some feedback. Use this feedback to correct common misconceptions along the way.

Some important points:

- Make sure the exams and the assignments (even homework) are *related to* stated objectives or outcomes. Students rebel (and they should!) against irrelevant "busy work."
- Pace the assignments and the exams so that you and the students get *early* and ongoing feedback. Don't schedule them so that all are due during the last week of class. It is too late then!

24. What should I do if a student is not doing well in my course?

This question underscores the need for early and ongoing evaluation of student learning. After returning an assignment or exam, invite students who did not do well to make an appointment to see you. (Make sure you included your office hours and location, phone number, and e-mail address on the syllabus.) Try to get the students to take this initiative. If they do not, then you call them!

During your meeting (individually and in private) use the steps of the nursing process:

- Assess what is going on and diagnose the problem. What variables are interfering with learning: poor study habits? poor time management? lack of motivation? fatigue? illness? a learning disability? Rarely is poor performance at the college level a factor of inadequate academic potential, but it can happen.
- Develop with the student some goals and a time line for reevaluation (short-term objectives are needed).
- Identify strategies/actions the student can take to remedy the problem. If there is a verified disability, get some help from your coordinator of services for persons with disabilities. All campuses receiving federal funds are required to have such an office.
- Evaluate again, early and ongoing.

25. How do I develop an exam?

Start with what is called an exam blueprint. Identify the learning objectives that the exam is to cover. Identify the amount of course content and how much time you needed to cover the content related to the identified objectives. (The more content and time, the more questions may be needed.) Remember, exam questions have to "fit." They have to be related to the learning objectives and the related course content.

Next decide on the format for the questions. The following formats are most frequently used:

- essay
- short answer and fill-in the blanks
- multiple choice
- true/false
- matching

In nursing, faculty primarily use multiple-choice questions because that is the format of NCLEX. Nursing courses that are clinically focused should have well-constructed multiple-choice questions that reflect steps of the nursing process (assessment, goals/objectives, interventions, evaluation). Questions should vary in their level of complexity (from recall to analysis to application, etc.). A general rule-of-thumb when determining how much testing time to allow is that students are allowed $1-1^1/_2$ minutes per multiple-choice question. This helps determine the number of questions for an exam, given the time constraints.

Some nursing courses, such as those dealing with issues and trends, may lend themselves to a variety of question formats (short answer, essay, as well as multiple choice). If feasible, you may want to use such variety in this situation so as to accommodate different test-taking skills of students. In any case, keep the exam reasonable in length and in level of complexity, and related to the learning objectives in the syllabus.

Developing good exam questions of any format is a sophisticated skill that requires a good tests and measurements course. If you have not taken one, it would be well worth your time and effort to take such a course. Meanwhile, you will find useful the instructor's manual and the test banks that accompany many texts.

26. What should I do if too many students fail an exam?

First, determine what constitutes "too many" students. If it is a well-designed exam with the proper mix of easy to difficult questions, it is quite possible that some students will not make the minimum passing grade. Remember the bell curve? If it appears that an inordinate number of students did not do well, several possibilities exist:

- The students were not well prepared for the exam. (Spring Block Party festivities were held just prior to the exam!)
- The exam covered material that was not emphasized in class or that the instructor simply did not present well.
- The exam questions were ambiguous and not well constructed.

There is not much you can do about the first possibility except to think about the exam schedule next time the course is taught. For the other two possibilities, you need to do some analysis:

- Check the match among the exam questions, the objectives, and the content. Is there a reasonably "good fit"?
- Review your class notes and teaching methods for the content covered by the exam.
- Was something going on to interfere with the teaching/learning process at that time?
- Do an item analysis of the questions. This is a strategy you will have learned in the tests and measurements course. If not, seek out a colleague who can teach you how it is done.

Pending the outcome of this review, you may want to make some adjustments if you find that the poor test results truly originated with you. This is a fairness issue and students are very tuned in to your sense of fairness. A word of caution—make sure that *you* were the problem before you make any adjustments. Do not capitulate to student requests for adjustments if they are not warranted. This is also a credibility issue. So, what kind of adjustments are we talking about?

- Worst-case scenario is to throw the whole exam out and start over after you have corrected the underlying problem(s). This is an extreme measure and a rarity.
- Most often, you can eliminate only the truly poor questions on the exam and recalculate the grades based on the valid questions that are left. "Valid" does not mean that all students answered the question correctly! An item analysis will help to tell you which questions were good and which ones were truly poor.

27. Should I go over the exam with the class after it is graded?

Most definitely, yes! Students need feedback and reviewing exams is a good teaching-learning strategy. Here are some important guidelines:

- Ahead of time, do your item analysis, see if any truly poor questions need to be examined, and adjust the point distribution accordingly.
- Determine ahead of time some areas that *you* want to address based on valid questions

that a number of the students missed.

- Distribute the exams and give the students a few minutes to look them over. Make sure the correct answers are somehow indicated for the students.
- Then, get the students' attention and announce those questions where *common* mistakes were made. It is *not* necessary to go over each and every question on an exam. Use this opportunity to briefly review or help students recall class content as rationale for the correct answers. If possible, indicate why the students' wrong answers were wrong. This helps students develop critical thinking.
- Announce to the class that you are available during office hours to meet individually with students who wish to ask about any particulars regarding their own exams.
- Do not get into "haggling" about points with the class. If a ground swell of concern occurs, tell the class that you will review their concerns and get back to them. (You'll need to go back to the test review process described in question 26.)

28. How do I grade written assignments?

Grading written assignments is facilitated if the written assignments are well-constructed in the first place. Written assignments have to be based on clear objectives. (There is that syllabus again!) Written assignments should certainly address course content, but also should be designed so that students are required to demonstrate critical thinking and written communication skills. The assignment can be constructed as a series of questions, or a series of "parts" for which you give instructions indicating what concepts, analysis, or synthesis the student should address in each part (e.g., "compare and contrast thus and such"). Indicate how many points each part is worth. Identify and state in the assignment the criteria you will be using when judging the students' responses in the parts of the paper. If proper sentence and paragraph structure, spelling, concept development, format (reference notes, margins, headings and title page, typos, etc.)— in short, if good writing skills are expected and part of the grading criteria—state in the assignment that "x number of points will be deducted from the grade for English and format errors." If students' late submission of the assignment will be penalized in the grading, state this as well.

Constructing the written assignment helps to objectify the grading even though subjectivity (your judgment) is part of the grading process. You need to have some reference points (criteria, standards) upon which to base your judgments.

Now, to the grading itself. Some faculty read all papers through once and then do a second, slower, deliberative reading. Although time-consuming, this is probably a good idea. During the second reading, make your judgments by comparing what the student wrote with the assignment directives and the criteria. Write comments reflecting your judgments on the students' papers. Remember, they need feedback. Make a determination regarding how many points the students' answers are worth for each part of the paper and write the point allocation on the paper. Your comments and point allocation have to be credible. Be prepared with an answer if the student asks, "Can you clarify your comments and justify the point allocation?" Do not forget to deduct points from the total if you said in the assignment that format and English count.

29. How do I calculate grades at the end of the semester?

How course grades will be calculated should have been stated in the course syllabus. The graded assignments and exams with their respective weighting need to be listed in the syllabus. If a minimum grade is required for the course to be counted toward degree requirements, it should be stated as well. At the end of the course, a student's grades for the respective assignments and exams get weighted and then added to constitute the course grade. The following example will demonstrate this:

Sample Grade Calculation

ITEM	GRADE	WEIGHT	CALCULATION	SCORE
Exam 1	70%	20%	70 x 0.20 =	14
Exam 2	78%	20%	78 x 0.20 =	15.6
Exam 3	82%	25%	82 x 0.25 =	20.5
Term paper	80%	25%	80 x 0.25 =	20
Homework	88%	10%	88 x 0.10 =	8.8

Course Grade = 78.9

Most colleges require final course grades to be reported as letter grades (A, B, C, etc.). To convert the student's final numerical grade (79%) to a letter grade requires that a prestated scale was delineated in the syllabus. Some institutions have a designated scale. Others allow respective departments to determine the scale of percent ranges for the different letter grades. In either case, the scales should be made known to the students, usually in the syllabus or a student handbook or both. An example follows:

Sample Scale of Percentage Grade to Letter Grade

% GRADE	LETTER GRADE
93-100	A
90 - 92	A-
86 - 89	B+
83 - 85	B
80 - 82	B-
76 - 79	C+
73 - 75	C
70 - 72	C-
66 - 69	D+
63 - 65	D
< 63	F

30. Should I curve grades?

Generally speaking, no. If you have constructed the course carefully in terms of objectives (outcomes) and teaching/learning strategies, and have used well-developed evaluation methods (tests, assignments) to measure student achievement (clear criteria), you should not have to curve grades. This assumes that you have developed reasonably good teaching methods and skills, too. Some view curving grades as a method for "rescuing" students on the lower end of the achievement scale. Maybe they should not be rescued. Remember, especially in the discipline of nursing, faculty have a responsibility to the public to graduate only those students who have achieved a safe level of competence.

31. If a student fails my course, does that mean that I do not know how to teach?

That is *not* a reasonable interpretation at all. Do not focus on the one student who failed and ignore the 99 others who passed the course! Laws of probability operate here, too. It is quite likely that some students may fail your course, and do not be surprised if that happens in an upper division course, too. While you may expect academically poor students to be "weeded out" in lower division courses, academically marginal students who "just made it through" those earlier courses may not be able to achieve the objectives of a higher level, more complex course.

Now, an inordinate number of failures in a course is another story. But that still does not mean you do not know how to teach. This case does warrant a thorough review, probably with the help of a mentor, of *all* aspects of the course, including:

- The general academic profile of the students in the class (as evidenced by prior achievement, standardized testing, etc.)
- The "personality" of the class. Classes do have personalities that emerge from the group dynamics. Sometimes there is an undercurrent of negative energy that may influence motivation and attitudes. Talk to colleagues who may have had this group of students in another course. What was their experience?
- Your performance from the development of the syllabus to the implementation of class lessons, exams, grading of assignments, etc. If you were monitoring your performance from day one of the course (see questions 23 and 24 above), you would be aware of problems in your performance and should have self-corrected those problems early enough to minimize the probability that student failure is your fault. It rarely is!

Remember, STUDENTS fail courses. FACULTY do not fail students.

32. What if a student thinks the grade he or she received in a course was unjustified or in error?

Most institutions have grade appeal policies and procedures that ensure due process for students who have grievances regarding their grades. If your institution or department does not have one, it would be a good idea to get them to develop one.

Grade appeal is a good safety net not only for students with legitimate concerns but also for faculty members who, after thorough review of alleged grading problems (see question 31), still conclude that the integrity of their course and grading procedures are intact. A grade appeal review will get at the truth and justice will prevail.

33. How can I tell if I am doing a good job in the classroom?

Just as students need feedback to learn, so also do faculty members need feedback to continue to develop as teachers. Some institutions have formal student evaluation processes for all courses. If your institution does not have one, you can (and should) develop your own. Some guidelines are:

- Safeguard the anonymity of the students doing the evaluations. No names. Have a student put completed forms in a sealed envelope and deliver them to a neutral party.
- This neutral party may compile the results for you, or hold the sealed envelope until after you submit your final course grades.
- Set the tone for the evaluations. Tell students that the purpose is to help improve education, particularly to give you help in improving your course and your teaching performance. Thank students for their input.
- Time the evaluation appropriately. To enhance the students' objectivity, you want to avoid doing the evaluations on an exam day or on the day you return exams or assignments. Assure the students that you will not look at the evaluations until after final course grades are submitted to the registrar.
- If you construct your own evaluation instrument, keep it easy to complete and score (a Likert scale works well). Include items about the course itself (e.g., course objectives and requirements were clear, the text was valuable, exams focused on material covered, course content was current, assignments and readings helped develop an understanding of course content). Also include items about your teaching performance (e.g., the instructor was knowledgeable, organized and well-prepared, paced presentation,

used resources effectively, encouraged thinking, encouraged questions, was punctual, returned exams and assignments promptly, was fair, was respectful to me, was available for office hours). Leave some room for and invite comments about the course and about you, the instructor.

• After you review the evaluations, *use* the feedback appropriately. With particularly negative feedback (and you will get some!), try to keep it in perspective, extract anything that can be used constructively, and then let go of it. With particularly positive feedback, "glow" awhile but then continue to build on those strengths. Do not get complacent! You are on the way to becoming a GREAT teacher!

BIBLIOGRAPHY

1. Billings DM, Halstead JA: Teaching in Nursing: A Guide for Faculty. Philadelphia, WB Saunders, 1998.
2. DePorter B, et al: Quantum Teaching: Orchestrating Student Success. Des Moines, Allyn & Bacon, 1999.
3. Haladyna TM: A Complete Guide to Student Grading. Des Moines, Allyn & Bacon, 1999.
4. Lyons RE, et al: The Adjunct Professor's Guide to Success: Surviving and Thriving in the College Classroom. Des Moines, Allyn & Bacon, 1999.
5. Oermann MH, Gaberson KB: Evaluation and Testing in Nursing Education. New York, Springer, 1998.
6. Schoenfeld AC, Magnan R: Mentor in a Manual: Climbing the Academic Ladder to Tenure, 2nd ed. Madison, WI, Magna, 1994.
7. Sudzina MR: Case Study Applications for Teacher Education: Cases of Teaching and Learning in the Content Areas. Des Moines, Allyn & Bacon, 1999.
8. Ulrich DL, Glendon KJ: Interactive Group Learning: Strategies for Nurse Educators. New York, Springer, 1999.

5. CLINICAL TEACHING

Priscilla L. Sagar, EdD, RN

1. What is my responsibility in the clinical area?

The instructor is responsible for the instruction and supervision of students in the clinical area. As such, the instructor is responsible for the provision of learning experiences that will facilitate (1) application and integration of theoretical concepts, (2) active participation and experience in patient care management, and (3) observation with active participation in professional roles for nurses in different settings. These activities are of the utmost importance and need to take place in the clinical setting so that students will truly be prepared to function as relevant and competent health care providers in a rapidly changing health care system.

Ensuring the safety of patients while facilitating students' learning are inherent responsibilities. The instructor is likewise responsible for the school's compliance with policies established by the clinical agency.

2. Who makes the arrangements for my clinical placement?

The school employing the instructor has written clinical affiliation agreements with clinical agencies. The actual placement itself has been selected by faculty after careful evaluation of agencies and their available units and patient population. Student and faculty evaluations from previous semesters should be reviewed to determine suitability of clinical settings.

The course faculty usually contacts the agency's Education Department or Staff Development Office to coordinate the placement. The faculty should confirm the clinical placement and arrange a planning meeting with the unit manager to discuss the educational objectives of the clinical experience prior to the actual clinical rotation. When the placement will be in a community agency, the faculty should arrange a meeting with the supervising nurse for discussion of educational objectives for the learning experience.

3. How do I know what my responsibility is to the clinical agency and the agency's responsibility to the students?

The written contract between the school and the agency specifies the responsibilities of clinical faculty to the agency as well as the agency's responsibilities to the students. Additionally, the school and the agency usually have policies delineating responsibilities of both parties. Frequently, the affiliation agreement specifies that instruction, evaluation, and administration of students are the responsibilities of the school, while the agency maintains full responsibility for patient care while providing learning experiences for students. It is helpful to clarify this at the outset.

4. I'm assigned to teach in a clinical agency that I am unfamiliar with. What should I do?

Schedule a planning meeting with the Education Department or Staff Development Office (or whoever is responsible for educational affiliations) and the unit manager of the specific unit for the clinical setting. In addition to discussing clinical objectives, students' learning needs, and clinical focus, arrange for your own orientation to the agency.

Orientation materials provided by the agency, such as checklists or self-learning modules, will be helpful. Other areas of importance include, but are not limited to, review of policy manuals and unit directives, unfamiliar equipment to be used by students in their patient care, documentation, and tour of all units involved. It will probably be helpful to arrange an observational experience in the agency during the hours that the clinical experience will occur. Such an experience enables faculty to gain a sense of the rhythm of the unit.

5. What should I include in the students' orientation to the clinical agency?

Review of the course's clinical objectives, focus, and method of student evaluation are a must. In addition, a discussion of the following areas is quite informative and may help alleviate student stresses about new clinical placement:

- Your expectations of students
- Expectations of students regarding the learning experience (this often encourages students to share their anxieties about the experience)
- Agency mission, goals, and philosophy of the agency's nursing department
- Students' learning needs and areas of interest (valuable information that will assist you in the selection of patients and learning experiences)
- "Mandatories," such as fire safety and a review of universal precautions (the agency may request written documentation that students have been oriented to this information)

A tour of the assigned unit and the hospital, including the cafeteria, is essential. Also, remember to tell students where they may leave their personal belongings and where clinical conferences will be held. One strategy that has been used successfully to orient students to the location of hospital departments, units, and supplies is a scavenger hunt. Give students a list of places and items to locate, allowing them to work in teams to find items on the list. Last but not least, do not forget to tell students where they should park if they provide their own transportation to the agency.

Clinical placement in community agencies requires additional information for students. If the clinical assignment is in a home care agency, students will need maps or directions to the patient's home. Also, it is wise to consider providing information regarding personal safety if students will be traveling to or through areas in which their personal safety might be threatened. Students also need specific instructions for contacting you (e.g., pager or cell phone number) if you will not be onsite during the clinical day.

6. How can I maintain good relationships with agency staff?

Collaboration, mutual respect, and open lines of communication between faculty, students, and agency staff are necessary ingredients for maintaining good relationships. Collaboration is a contributive, ongoing partnership between professionals which enables problem solving. Mutual respect between faculty, students, and staff involves esteem for each other's humanity and expertise. Appreciate the fact that staff are often overworked and burdened with concerns unrelated to your presence in the agency. Open lines of communication will prevent conflict and confusion about the objectives and goals for the rotation and the priorities and protocols that the staff adapts to accommodate student learning experiences. Seek staff input regarding students' activities (i.e., how is their presence in the agency perceived by staff?) and address staff concerns immediately.

7. When and how should I select patients for the students?

Class and clinical objectives for the course, weekly clinical focus, and student competencies and learning needs are salient points to consider in planning what patients to select for the students. In advanced nursing courses, a student survey of past clinical experiences and special areas of interest will be beneficial in the selection of patients.

First, the "when." Depending on the time of day of the clinical experience and your expectations for students' preparation prior to clinical, you may want to prepare students' clinical assignments the day before the experience or just prior to the experience.

If you expect students to review charts prior to the experience, then you will probably want to post the assignment the day before clinical. On the other hand, if your routine is for students to receive their assignments when they arrive for clinical, then you might wait until just before the clinical experience begins to select patients or other clinical activities. If you prepare the assignment the day prior to the clinical experience, it is a good idea to identify alternative patients for students in the event that the patients you selected are no longer available on the clinical day. This saves valuable clinical time when the need to change student assignments arises because of patient transfer, discharges, expiration, or refusal. You will probably want to allow at least an hour and a half to review patient charts and other information that will enable you to select appropriate learning experiences.

Now, the "how." Allow plenty of time for this project, especially at the beginning of the semester until you become more familiar with the unit or agency. Generally speaking, students can integrate theoretical concepts better when the clinical experiences are closer in time to the discussion of concepts in the classroom. Begin the selection process by familiarizing yourself with the patients on the unit or in the community agency. If some students will rotate to other areas of the hospital (such as the operating room) or another agency, plan a rotation schedule. Talk to the nurses and let them know what type of learning experiences you are looking for. Review your list of student learning needs (gathered during the orientation to the agency). Decide which type of experiences you want for each student. If you select patients because their care will provide valuable experience with psychomotor skills (respiratory suctioning, urinary catheterization, dressing change, etc.), you may need to perform the actual procedure yourself, explaining your actions to the student and encouraging the student to assist if the student has not learned the skill in the classroom or college lab. Students may then be allowed to perform the procedure after a successful return demonstration in the lab.

Proponents of this practice believe that when the learning experience outweighs the amount of time spent with a few of the students teaching a new skill, it is more advisable that the experience is assigned to the student(s). The opportunity for certain learning experiences occurs infrequently and may not be available to the students later in the course of their education. So, be flexible and take advantage of valuable learning experiences as they occur.

The disadvantage of assigning students to patients with current or anticipated procedures that students have not had ample time to practice in the clinical laboratory is that additional faculty time to teach and demonstrate skills in the clinical setting is required, thus taking time away from other learning experiences.

When assigning students to administer medications, keep in mind students' competence with medication administration. Beginning students can take an inordinate amount of time to prepare and administer medications for one patient! Assigning too many beginning students to prepare and administer medications may result in late administration of medications and a frazzled faculty member who spends the clinical day supervising medication experiences. Remember, you need to allow time to supervise and teach those students who are not preparing medications, too. Therefore, if you have a group of beginning students, consider assigning medication administration to only a few of the students rather than involving the whole group.

It is crucial to remember that students should only be assigned to provide care which they are competent to administer. Patient safety always takes precedence over student learning.

8. How do I plan the students' clinical day?

Plan learning activities according to the students' level within the nursing program, weekly clinical focus, amount of supervision the students will need, and the type and acuity of patients in the unit or agency. In addition, investigate other learning activities in the unit or the institution as a whole, such as nursing rounds, conferences, and meetings of other relevant groups.

Include pre- and post-conferences in planning the day, although sometimes it may not be possible to have a conference due to time constraints. Remember that flexibility is the key. Faculty must be flexible enough to use alternative learning experience as they arise.

9. What is pre- and post-conference?

Lasting about an hour, the pre-conference is a planning discussion preceding the clinical experience. The pre-conference is used for (1) directing learning for the day as per the clinical focus, (2) integrating the nursing process in client care, and (3) laying the foundation for evaluation and analysis during post-conference. Both the instructor and the students must come prepared for pre-conference. Be certain to answer students' questions and to evaluate the students' abilities to provide care safely. For example, if the student is assigned to perform a fingerstick glucose, ascertain that the student knows when to do it, what the normal parameters are, and what to do if the result is abnormal.

Post-conference is, ideally, held immediately after the clinical experience. Its purpose is to analyze and evaluate patient care. Due to time constraints, the post-conference can be done effectively in a shorter period of time than pre-conference. The faculty role is to act as a facilitator and motivator, encouraging creative thought and multiple perspectives from all students.

Clinical conferences serve as an excellent learning environment, cultivating the leadership abilities and critical thinking skills of students. Students should be encouraged to share patient care problems and use the scientific method to arrive at possible solutions.

10. How will the staff know exactly what the students will be doing?

During the planning meeting with the agency, discuss the clinical objectives for the rotation as well as the program level of the students and their learning needs. Some agencies have several affiliating schools or different levels of students from the same school. Clarifications like these minimize confusion in terms of roles and expectations.

Specifically, the staff will be more aware of students' clinical activities if the instructor discusses the student assignment with the nurse in charge, posts clinical assignments in the unit or agency, delineating each student's activities, and encourages every student to discuss activities for the day with the primary nurse as early as possible during the shift. Notes clipped on the medication kardex specifying which medications will be given by students will help remind the staff during the course of the day not to administer the medications to the patients.

11. How can I supervise all the students in my clinical group?

This is one of the biggest challenges in clinical teaching! A clinical group may have anywhere from 7 to 10 students, with most schools and agencies placing the cap at 10 students. While it is not easy to supervise that many students in a clinical group, the following strategies will be helpful:

- Rotate students for a day or two in special areas like the operating room, x-ray, or ambulatory surgery.
- Assign a student as clinical coordinator for the day; this student will assist and supervise the other students with the instructor.
- Pair students in dyads to manage care for complex patients.

Assignments in special areas give students a chance to integrate physical and psychosocial care of patients undergoing special procedures into the total care of the patient. The student experience as clinical coordinator is an ideal chance to collaborate with classmates and other health team members in patient care management and to cultivate leadership potential among nursing students. Students working in pairs learn from collaboration with each other and generally find the experience less stressful.

12. How do I allocate my time among students in my clinical group?
An instructor can allocate his or her time among students by spending more time with three or four students per day and then doing the same with others the following clinical day. This works as well when performing procedures with students such as physical assessment and medication administration. Both assignments require the integration of cognitive, psychomotor, and affective domains of learning and, hence, require more time, especially for beginning students.

It goes without saying that it is better to work with fewer students than to feel rushed supervising and teaching them, which will likely cause added anxiety and stress for students and faculty. This is worthy of faculty consideration, since clinical itself creates varying degrees of stress for students. Numerous studies have documented student stress in the clinical setting. However, the stress of faculty has not been explored.

Remember, you are responsible for all students in your clinical group, so emphasize with students the need to seek you out if they are unsure about performing a particular activity or if they suspect a change in the patient's condition. It can be very unsettling for faculty to be involved with one or a few students, while wondering what the remaining students are doing! Developing a good rapport with students will encourage them to seek you out for questions and concerns.

13. How do I know what the other students are doing if I am busy with one or two students?
You might want to do a quick round of the unit whenever it is possible to safely leave the one or two students for a few minutes. This will enable you to assess the situation with the rest of the group. Sometimes it is not always possible to know what the rest of the group is doing, such as when you are supervising a student who is performing care for a patient in strict isolation. Strategies suggested in question 11 might be employed here. The bottom line is that, no matter how efficient you are as a clinical instructor, you will not know what every student is doing every minute! This underscores the need for developing a good rapport with students and making your expectations known (for not undertaking anything for which they have not previously been given the "go ahead" by you).

14. How do I teach students critical thinking in the clinical setting?
Critical thinking is the ability to arrive at sensible, judicious decisions in carrying out the nursing care of patients. In the clinical setting, the use of case studies and case method, discussions, and written assignments can be used to teach critical thinking. Case studies provide opportunities for students to perceive problems, identify multiple possible solutions, and arrive at logical conclusions. Discussion, done individually or with small groups of students, facilitate problem-solving and decision-making. Written assignments about problems and issues in clinical practice, along with critiques and personal stance on those issues, provide students avenues to think critically. Asking students to provide rationale for their decisions and actions facilitates critical thinking. So, select one or two interesting patients each day and use the case method to structure the discussion.

15. What should I do if students ask me something that I don't know the answer to?
You do not need to be the "sage on a stage," but rather a facilitator of learning. It is impossible for anyone to know everything. In that instance, you and the student(s) can con-

sult references together to find the answer to the question. Alternatively, assign the search for an answer as a mutual assignment for yourself and student for the next clinical day.

It is appropriate to point out that the rapid explosion of technology and scientific information may change current practice, and that nurses need to update their knowledge continuously. Nurses who are experts in specific fields may be novices in others, hence reinforcing the need for collaboration between nurses in practice, as well as with those in education and research. Ideally, nursing educators will engage in practice and research concurrently.

16. What should I do if a student makes a mistake?

You are responsible for intervening in situations where the consequences of a student error will harm the patient. Otherwise, mistakes are part of the learning process. A learning environment laden with trust and mutual respect between students and faculty is conducive to the admission of error, seeking feedback to remedy the situation, and valuing the learning from the incident.

In case of a medication error, you, the student, and the patient's nurse should consult with the physician to rectify the error and ensure patient safety. Appropriate documentation protocol about the incident is followed. Encourage the student to reflect on the possible factors that contributed to the error and the actions needed to avoid similar situations in the future.

17. How do I make sure that students provide all the care they have been assigned to do and still end clinical on time?

To end the clinical experience on time, resist the temptation to schedule too many special assignments for the day. The time for ending the clinical day should be scheduled at least 30 minutes before the actual end of the day to allow for unavoidable delays. Otherwise, time for scheduled post-conference at the end of the clinical experience will be lost due to a lack of time.

Sometimes it is not possible for students to perform all of the assigned care due to a change in the patient's condition, diagnostic tests, or other conditions that are beyond the control of you or the students. However, if the student did not complete the assignment due to poor organization skills, you will need to provide appropriate feedback and recommendations to the student to enhance organizational skills. Any aspect of patient care which was not completed must be reported by the student to the primary nurse.

18. What should I do if I think a student is cutting corners with patient care?

It is imperative to supervise the student closely if you suspect this has occurred. You can follow-up with the patient regarding care provided, such as physical assessment after a bath, or ask the patient to verbalize what he or she has learned after a teaching session by the student. These strategies might be helpful in assessing whether patient care has been performed according to standards.

It is necessary to schedule an individual counseling session with the student if care has been purposefully omitted or if the student's care is deemed to be below standards. The discussion and documentation must clearly state what the student needs to do to meet standards, the time frame involved, the student's plan for meeting the objectives, and the consequences if the situation does not improve to your satisfaction.

19. What should I do with the student who is overly anxious in clinical?

Many students find clinical stressful and experience anxiety that interferes with clinical performance. When a student is overly anxious, assess the sources of anxiety and explore possible solutions with the student. If the anxiety is about the new rotation or skills required, advising the student to practice in the skills lab and/or increasing familiarity with the clinical agency will probably lessen the anxiety. It might help to give less complex patient assignments to the student for the first two weeks of clinical. Once the student experiences success with managing the clinical assignment, the stress and anxiety should lessen. If not, the student may have a more serious problem that warrants professional counseling. Refer the student to the college counseling center.

20. How do I handle the student who is very slow and unable to finish his/her assignment?

Work closely with the student to determine the student's ability to prioritize care and plan for the entire day. Assess the student's performance of assigned activities. Is there an attempt at perfectionism? Does the student need more practice in the skills lab to enhance skills and, hence, self-confidence? Or, worse yet, is the student just slow with activities in general, in and out of the clinical setting? Ask the student his or her perception of the problem. Advising the student to develop a written timetable to use as a guide during the clinical day may provide the needed structure for the student to complete the assignment on time. Instruct the student to spend time in the skills lab if he or she needs more practice with selected psychomotor skills. If the student's inexperience is a contributing factor, the problem should resolve as the student progresses through the course.

21. What should I do if a student performs at an unsafe level?

All students need ongoing feedback about their clinical performance. The unsafe student's performance needs to be discussed privately with the student, with written documentation completed regularly during the course. Documentation should clearly describe the unsafe practice, the objective(s) not met, and the actual consequences to the patient. If the school has a provision for written developmental contracts in situations such as this, the contract should include the following:

- A description of the unsafe practice
- Objective(s) not met
- Actual or potential consequences of the unsafe actions
- Desired performance
- Time frame the student has to meet the objective(s)
- Consequences if the student does not meet the objective(s)
- Student's comments

Suspension from clinical or other academic or disciplinary action will depend upon how many other times the student has performed at an unsafe level in the past and whether the school has clearly written protocol about unsafe performance. If the student performs unsafely at the time of the summative evaluation (done at the end of the course), the student fails the clinical component of the course. If the course is structured so that a passing grade in the course is dependent upon a passing grade in the clinical lab, the student would then fail the entire course.

22. A student has good technical skills but does not answer my questions satisfactorily. What does this mean and how should I handle it?

Explore the possible reason for the inability to answer the questions satisfactorily. Possible reasons here could be poorly organized thinking processes resulting in a poor articulation of the answer, increased anxiety in a new rotation, or lack of preparation, to name a few. Discussion with the student to explore this problem will, hopefully, provide some insights that will be helpful to the student and you. Feedback to the student must include positive remarks about the psychomotor skills and the encouragement to further work on the ability to articulate theoretical concepts. If the student cannot answer questions correctly due to the lack of critical thinking skills, it is likely that the student will have difficulty with other aspects of the course.

23. What should I do when the staff delivers patient care in a way that is incongruent with that which students are taught?

It depends upon whether or not the incongruence violates the patient's rights to safe, competent care. If the care is a creative, alternate way for an intervention, this is a chance for students to see multiple application of concepts in the clinical setting. If the patient care does not meet accepted standards, then faculty must discuss this with the staff nurse and the charge nurse. If the issue is not resolved at this level, the director of staff development and the director of nursing for the clinical agency should be notified.

24. I don't know how to operate all the equipment in the clinical setting. Is it appropriate to ask the staff to demonstrate to the students and me?

It is a good idea to spend a day or two on the unit, prior to the first clinical day, to orient yourself to the unit and specialized equipment used on the unit. Of course, there may still be occasions when you are unfamiliar with equipment. It is appropriate to ask one of the staff nurses to demonstrate the equipment to you and the students, provided you can be flexible about the "when." Staff nurses are usually pleased to have a teaching role for faculty and students, provided it does not interfere with their work. Occasionally making a request for a "mini" instruction session sends the message that you respect the staff's knowledge and skill.

25. Sometimes it seems as though staff perceives students as being in the way. How should I handle that?

It would be helpful to validate this perception with the staff. If your perception is valid, try to delineate specific times. Perhaps students are crowding the nurses' station while they read charts. If students are "hanging out" in the nurses' station after they finish patient care, refer back to your expectations for students. Do you expect them to demonstrate initiative and seek out their own learning experiences? If not, perhaps you should rethink this.

Sometimes students have a tendency to direct all of their questions to the staff instead of you. If they frequently interrupt staff while they are busy, staff might readily perceive them as being in the way and wonder what your role is. Make it clear to students when they should seek you out with their questions and when it is acceptable to seek out staff. There is a fine line between encouraging collegiality between students and staff and facilitating bothersome behavior!

If the unit is small, and students really do need a place to review charts and document their care, or confer with each other or you, perhaps you could find an empty room for this purpose. Just be sure to remind students to let staff know when they remove charts from the nurses' station.

Finally, if the student group is large, remember the strategies in question 11.

26. The unit is so busy. I feel that we are in the way. What should I do?

If it is not possible to assign the students individually, or in pairs, with a nurse so that the students can actively participate in the care of patients, then it might be helpful to start a post-conference a bit early. You might focus on a discussion of what is happening on the unit, the day's learning activities and students' interventions, presentation of case studies, or viewing a relevant videotape. These activities might be more meaningful to the students and facilitate more learning than remaining on a busy unit where students perceive that they are interfering with the rhythm of the unit. On the other hand, being participants in a busy unit may give students a sense of accomplishment, mastery, and reality in health care.

Much will depend on the experience of the students. Beginning students who normally take longer periods of time to accomplish simple activities may not be ready to participate on a unit that is very busy. Experienced students might be a welcome relief to staff since their presence allows staff to focus on other patients. Of course, if the unit is always very busy and you always feel that students are interfering with the process of patient care, validate your perceptions with the staff; you may need to rethink your decision to place students on this unit. Keep in mind, though, that high acuity and overburdened staff are realities in today's health care environment. You may need to find innovative ways to enable students to meet learning objectives in a high-acuity environment.

27. Certain staff members do not want students to do anything except observe their patients. What should I do?

This situation reinforces the need to meet with the unit manager, and even staff, prior to the students' first day on the unit, to share your expectations and the clinical objectives. If you have already done this and staff are still reluctant to let students provide patient care, it is time to speak with the head nurse and the staff again about the need for students to actively participate in patient care. Try to find out why the nurse(s) do not want students to provide care. Perhaps they have had previous negative experiences with students or lack confidence in your ability to supervise the students. If the problem is not remedied, a discussion with the coordinator of student placements at the institution is warranted. If these approaches do not work, perhaps you could select patients who are assigned to more cooperative staff. Finally, if all efforts to promote student participation in patient care are unsuccessful, you will probably want to recommend that the school not seek affiliation with this unit in the future.

28. How should I grade students' clinical performance?

First, learn your school's policy for grading clinical performance. Most schools use some sort of a checklist. Clinical evaluation instruments vary considerably, with some schools using the same instrument for all courses and other schools using evaluation instruments developed by faculty teaching the course. Regardless of which type of evaluation instrument is used by your school, the instrument should be closely related to clinical and course objectives. Moreover, the evaluation instrument should be valid and reliable, as well as sensitive enough to distinguish between the clinically strong student and the weak student.

Depending upon your school's policy, a final clinical grade of pass/fail or a letter grade will be assigned. Questions that should be answered include determining when you should evaluate the student. Is evaluation an ongoing process based upon a pattern of performance, or are there certain days that are identified as evaluation days? Ideally, faculty will give students ongoing verbal feedback regarding their performance. A written midterm evaluation, although formative in nature, provides documentation of the student's performance at that time. Likewise, a midterm evaluation provides an opportunity for the faculty to meet with each student individually to review progress and learning needs. Be sure to note each student's strengths as well as weaknesses. When you provide feedback to the student, it is a good idea to tell the student first what he or she does well. Then you can proceed to identify areas where improvement is needed. Remember to be specific with your feedback, so the student knows exactly where he or she needs to improve.

29. What are anecdotal notes and how are they used?

Anecdotal notes are your daily or weekly notes regarding the student's performance for that day or week. A daily anecdotal sheet/checklist that students sign and add comments to is helpful in keeping track of student performance. Anecdotal notes may or may not be filed with the student's clinical evaluation instrument at the conclusion of the semester. Even if anecdotal notes do not become a part of the student's file, it is important to remember that they are student records and may be subpoenaed in court. If you keep anecdotal notes, keep them on all students, not just on those students who are having difficulty. Moreover, record both strengths and weakness. Keeping anecdotal notes only on weaker students and recording only deficiencies may invite charges of discrimination should a grade dispute arise.

30. What should I do if a student is failing clinical?

An interesting question. First and foremost, remember that clinical is a learning experience. Keeping this in mind, avoid the temptation to classify a student as passing or failing until the semester ends. Remember, students learn at different rates, and the late bloomer may still be able to meet the clinical objectives by the end of the semester.

Since you will be providing feedback to students on an ongoing basis, the goal is that students will incorporate your feedback and move toward achievement of the clinical objectives. Students may either progress toward this goal or not. However, labeling a student as failing prior to the end of the semester may invite a self-fulfilling prophecy. Therefore, until the course ends, no student should be classified as failing. This does not mean that you withhold information from students regarding their performance. As noted in the previous question, ongoing feedback is vital to the students' learning.

Students who are not meeting clinical objectives need to be aware of this as early as possible. Individual conferences are needed where there is written documentation of objectives not being met, including specific instances where students did not meet the objectives. Provide clear statements of what the student needs to do and how much time the student has to achieve the objectives. The student, likewise, should state in writing how he or she plans to achieve the objectives. Developing a formal contract with the student, which is attached to the clinical evaluation form, is a useful strategy.

31. I will be teaching a community-based clinical course. How do I keep track of what students are doing when I cannot be with them all of the time?

Site visits are very important in a community-based clinical course. The following strategies will be helpful in keeping track of what students are doing:

• Observe as many activities as possible that students participate in.
• Talk to each nurse who had an opportunity to work with the students.
• Schedule one or more home visits with each student and their primary nurse.

The frequency of agency and home visits will depend upon the number of students in the clinical group, the distance between the clinical sites, and the length of the clinical day. Since students are often assigned individually to a clinical site, you may find that you have students in as many as 8 or 10 clinical sites on any clinical day. When you are not present at a clinical site with the student, there should be an efficient and effective method for students to contact you if they have questions or need help. Many faculty carry pocket pagers or cell phones for this purpose.

BIBLIOGRAPHY

1. Alexander MF: Integration of clinical and theoretical teaching. In Modly DM, Zanotti R, Poletti P, Fitzpatrick JJ (eds): Advancing Nursing Education Worldwide. New York, Springer, 1995, pp 81-98.
2. Bradshaw MJ: Philosophical approaches to clinical instruction. In Fuszard B (ed): Innovative Teaching Strategies in Nursing. Gaithersburg, MD, Aspen, 1995, pp 216-211.
3. Carpenito LJ, Duespohl TA: A Guide for Effective Clinical Instruction. Rockville, MD, Aspen, 1981.
4. Christensen P: Issues in clinical teaching: Cautionary tales for nursing faculty. In Fuszard B (ed): Innovative Teaching Strategies in Nursing. Gaithersburg, MD, Aspen, 1995, pp 294-302.
5. Conger MM, Mezza I: Fostering critical thinking in nursing students in the clinical setting. Nurse Educator 21:11-15, 1996.
6. Massarweh LJ: Promoting a positive clinical experience. Nurse Educator 24:44-47, 1999.
7. Musinski B: The educator as facilitator: A new kind of leadership. Nursing Forum 34:23-29, 1999.
8. Oermann MH, Gaberson KB: Evaluation and Testing in Nursing Education. New York, Springer, 1998.
9. Reilly DE, Oermann MH: Clinical Teaching in Nursing Education. New York, National League for Nursing, 1992.
10. Weingarten CT: The role of faculty in developing leadership in students. In Andersen CAF (ed): Nursing Student to Nursing Leader: The Critical Path to Leadership Development. Albany, New York, Delmar, 1999, pp 87-106.

6. RESEARCH AND SCHOLARSHIP

Dolores A. Bower, PhD, RN, and Bernadette D. Curry, PhD, RN

1. What is research?

In the nursing faculty role, research can be defined in several ways. It can be related to testing a theory, such as Roy's Adaptation Model, or anchored in a special clinical area of practice, such as gerontological nursing. Its focus might relate to broad professional issues, such as the public perception of the nurse role, or may be based in developing models of health care delivery. Research is purposeful inquiry into a particular question or "problem." It is a process that begins with identification of a problem statement, involves data collection and analysis, and concludes with some form of dissemination. When research is an expectation of the faculty role, the academic institution may provide further definition of research that reflects its mission.

2. Does research differ from scholarship?

Scholarship is a broad, all-encompassing term, which includes the conduct of research. The American Association of Colleges of Nursing 1999 position statement defines nursing scholarship as those activities that advance the teaching, research, and practice of nursing through rigorous inquiry that is:
- Significant to the profession
- Creative
- Able to be documented
- Able to be replicated or elaborated upon
- Able to be peer-reviewed[5]

Scholarship takes a holistic form and embraces many processes, including professional writing, presenting, mentoring, collaborating, and the art and science of teaching. Despite these differences, the terms research and scholarship are often used interchangeably in academic settings.

3. Why are research and scholarship important?

According to Boyer, scholarly activities enable the discipline and the participants to be "intellectually alive." Scholarly activities motivate faculty and create excitement in the lecture halls and clinical laboratories. Both research and scholarship are essential to a profession, particularly a practice profession such as nursing. As leaders in their discipline, nurse faculty contribute to the knowledge base in professional nursing through their research.

4. Are research and scholarship more important than teaching, advisement, and community service?

No, but that depends on the type of academic institution and its mission. Typically, liberal arts colleges emphasize teaching, advisement, and service, whereas a large public research institution with graduate programs may place research on a par with teaching and service. Most institutions will expect faculty involvement in all areas: research, teaching, advisement, and service, but the emphasis on the components will vary.

5. What is expected of me in this area?

The novice faculty member needs to determine the emphasis that is placed on various workload components and on promotion and tenure. At the time of your appointment, faculty orientation should clarify these aspects of the job. Regardless of the particular emphasis that individual institutions may place on the components, it is widely accepted that research and scholarly activities enhance all aspects of the faculty role, especially the teaching role.

6. How much time should I devote to scholarly activities?

A general rule of thumb is to apportion your time according to the expectations for your faculty role. For example, if the major emphasis at your institution is on teaching, the majority of your time should be devoted to strategies and techniques in teaching. However, if faculty are expected to have refereed publications and/or externally funded research, the expectation is substantial. To calculate a rough proportion, take the criteria for promotion and tenure and determine the weighting. Once that proportion is known, the next step is to compute the total hours in your work week. An example is a weighting of 60% teaching, 30% scholarly activities, and 10% service. If your work week is estimated to be 50 hours, then 30 hours will be devoted to teaching activities, 15 hours to scholarly activities, and 5 hours per week to service. Some faculty who have 9- or 10-month academic year appointments will use the summer months for scholarly activities and the academic months for teaching and service.

7. How do I fit research and scholarship in my workload?

There is no *one* way to do this. The overall plan should be based on a 3–5-year interval, typically the probationary time prior to evaluation for tenure. In a multi-year plan, the first year may include a smaller proportion of time for scholarship compared to the third year.

Faculty may wish to negotiate for "release time" for research. This means that teaching assignments or service to the college or university may be reduced so that faculty time can be devoted to research. The likelihood of negotiating release time depends on the mission of the university.

The decision to blend research into the week's activities depends upon the topic or area of scholarly work. For example, if the research is closely related to the area in which you teach (in the classroom or clinical), it may be comfortable and appropriate to allocate time each week to work on a proposal, report, or manuscript. Many faculty will try to carve out a day each week, and zealously guard that time, for their scholarly work. The ideal arrangement for efficient management of time is to blend the area of research with practice, teaching, and service. Keeping current in one's area will benefit all aspects of the role.

8. How do I get started with writing?

Though it may seem obvious, the first step in writing is having something to write about. Publications usually stem from research findings that need to be reported. Many publications, however, may originate from other aspects of your faculty role, such as determining new protocols, elaborating on a curriculum decision, or reporting on an innovative teaching strategy. These "academic or practice experiences" often require a search of the literature, interpretation, and analysis. Frequently, faculty may take on a task to better understand an existing problem and conclude with findings that they wish to share with others. These "task force" or committee opportunities often will involve a group, resulting in a multi-authored publication.

9. Is it better to consider single-authored publications?

It depends. Some criteria for faculty require single versus coauthored publications, believing that the former is more scholarly and reflective of the individual's work. The decision to consider coauthoring, then, may be simply a personal preference. It is generally considered an advantage for a novice to coauthor, being mentored, while contributing to the manuscript. Coauthoring can be a good idea if authors wish to complement their style, work patterns, and/or areas of expertise. Some individuals find it helpful to keep to a schedule and deadlines if they work with another person. Regardless of how you choose to work, the steps in identifying an appropriate journal, obtaining author guidelines, and proceeding are the same.

If faculty decide to collaborate in writing an article for publication, it is essential to establish some ground rules prior to entering an agreement. Regardless of the relationship between colleagues, agreements regarding first author, timelines, and work division should be formal and clear.

10. How do I go about publishing my work?

One of the first steps is to identify a suitable forum/journal for your manuscript ideas. It is important to identify the journal prior to developing the manuscript, as each journal may have a particular style, format, and other requirements. By perusing potential journals, you will quickly determine whether your topic is an appropriate match. For example, some journals will only consider research-based manuscripts. Once you have identified some likely journals, the next step is obtaining the guidelines for authors. They can usually be found in the front or back of the journal, and will also indicate whether a query letter or entire manuscripts are invited. The guidelines will also describe the type of article that will be considered, writing style, and review process.

Once you have submitted a manuscript for review, you must wait until the review process is completed prior to submitting to another journal. In other words, you cannot submit the same manuscript to multiple journals at the same time. Review processes can take from 2-6 months. If you are considering several journals, it would make sense to submit first to the journal that has the shortest review process. It is unusual to have a manuscript accepted without any modifications, especially for the novice writer. If you receive feedback with specific reviewer comments, you will want to seriously consider responding to the reviewer notes and resubmitting the manuscript. The reviewer will usually state explicitly if the manuscript is not suited to the journal.

11. What are refereed journals or presentations?

A refereed publication or presentation is one that undergoes a review process and selection. The manuscript or proposal is held up to standards and meets a professional level of scholarship. If not stated explicitly, a journal is refereed when the review process includes peer reviewers or editorial boards.

12. How much time should I allow for publication of a manuscript?

Though it may vary by journal, the entire process from identifying a topic, drafting the manuscript outline, identifying the appropriate journal, and the review process may take 12–16 months or longer. If the manuscript is rejected by one journal, a second (or even third journal submission) will extend the time.

13. Are there costs associated with scholarly activities?

There are no fees associated with publication of manuscripts for most nursing journals; however, some medical journals charge the author a fee for publication. Even though the journal may not charge a fee for publication, the author might incur costs related to literature searches, manuscript preparation, permission to use copyrighted material, and duplication.

Research, on the other hand, can be very costly to conduct. The cost may be in terms of both time and resources. Since the conduct of research can be costly to a faculty member, "seed money" or "start-up funds" may be available within the institution to offset initial expense. When the costs related to scope of research, sample, intervention, or data collection are substantial, faculty may seek external funds from foundations, professional organizations, or federal agencies. Whether competing for internal or external funds, all research proposals undergo some peer review, and the process is very competitive.

14. What does "publish or perish" mean?

This is a phrase that captures the importance of scholarly activities in academe. It specifically refers to the publishing expectation for promotion in rank and tenure.

BIBLIOGRAPHY

1. American Association of Colleges of Nursing: Position Statement: Defining Scholarship for the Discipline of Nursing. Washington, DC; 1999.
2. Baughman J, Goldman K : College ranking and faculty publications. Change 31:44-51, 1999.
3. Boyer E: Scholarship Reconsidered: Priorities of the Professoriate. Princeton, NJ, The Carnegie Foundation for the Advancement of Teaching, 1990.
4. Brown SA et al: Nursing Perspective of Boyer's Scholarship Paradigm. Nurse Educator 20: 26-30, 1995.
5. Colbeck CL: Merging in a seamless blend: how faculty integrate teaching and research. J Higher Educ 69:647-58, 1998.
6. Fondiller S: The Writer's Workbook: Health Professionals' Guide to Getting Published. Sudbury, MA, Jones & Bartlett Publishers, 1999.
7. Ruby J: History of higher education: Educational reform and the emergence of nursing professoriate. J Nurs Educ 38: 23-27, 1999.

7. FACULTY SERVICE ACTIVITIES

Victoria Rizzo Nikou, PhD, RN, CS

1. What is meant by service?

Faculty service is defined as offering professional contributions on a voluntary basis. The faculty member does not receive monetary compensation for these contributions. Service activities include those to the college or university, the community, and the profession.

2. Why is service important to the faculty role?

Since the early days of academe, service has been an important component in the triad of professional behaviors that form the core of faculty role expectations. Service is necessary at the college/university level, since it sets the standards for policies, requirements, and curricular issues. Role modeling and mentoring are important expectations for educators; it is through service activities related to student organizations and committees that students have the opportunity to observe and collaborate with faculty members. Florence Nightingale also spoke of the need for the professional nurse to engage in community service. Service activities enable the professional to offer significant contributions to their communities of interest.

3. What types of service activities are faculty expected to pursue?

Faculty are expected to provide service in three areas: to the college or university, to the profession, and to the community.

College or university service generally includes activities that contribute to decision making and policy formation for the institution, as well as activities, excluding teaching and research, that enable the college or university to meet its mission. Examples include:
- Participation on department, school, and university-wide committees
- Chairing committees
- Participation on *ad hoc* committees and task forces
- Chairing the department or division
- Sharing one's expertise within the college through the presentation of workshops or lectures, or by leading a discussion forum
- Advising student organizations
- Academic advisement

Professional service encompasses service to professional nursing or educational organizations at the local, regional, national, and/or international level(s). Generally speaking, the higher the level, the more prestigious the service. Examples include:
- Holding office in a professional organization at the local, regional, or national level
- Chairing committees within professional organizations
- Contributing to organizational policy formation
- Serving as a site visitor for the CCNE, NLNAC, or regional accreditor
- Serving on the governing board of a nursing program or regional accreditor

Community (public) service offers a broad array of opportunities for the nurse faculty member. Examples include:

- Consultation
- Serving on the governing board of a community organization
- Offering community education programs
- Public speaking in your area of expertise
- Contributing to public policy formation
- Testifying before governmental bodies

4. I am not clear on community service—elaborate, please!

Faculty are often concerned about how much or what type of community involvement is considered service. For example, if I belong to a church, community service organization, or PTA, does that count? Generally, if your only involvement is membership, then the answer is no. However, if you provide leadership by lending your professional expertise to the activities of the group, then it is probably a service activity. Some specific examples of service activities are listed in the table below.

GENERAL AREA OF SERVICE	SPECIFIC EXAMPLE
Serving as a member of chair of a community board or one of its committees	Serving as chairperson of the Health and Human Services Committee
Organizing a grassroots task force, coalition, committee, or health fair	Organizing a grassroots task force to examine teenage suicide or child abuse in your community
Speaking on health-related issues for a community group	Teaching Boy Scouts and Girl Scouts about riding safely in automobiles or teaching a senior citizen group in a church about taking medications safely
Serving on a subcommittee for a local chapter of a national community health organization such as the American Cancer Society or the American Heart Association	Serving on the nursing education subcommittee of your local chapter of the American Cancer Society
Volunteering to solicit funds from the community for one of these organizations	Contacting potential corporate donors or collecting monies door-to-door in your community
Serving as a member of a board of directors for local nursing homes, senior or youth centers, or other reputable community organizations	Serving as a board member of Big Brothers/ Big Sisters
Lobbying for the public's welfare	Meeting with state legislators to garner support for a change in drinking and driving laws or meeting with local legislators to garner support for helmet laws

Innovative examples of service include offering contributions through the print and broadcast media. In some localities, nurses have been able to initiate radio and cable television programs on a weekly or monthly basis or participate in public service announcement segments. Advice columns, questions and answer segments, and editorials are fine examples of service through print media.

Personal examples by this writer of community service that have been gratifying and valued by the community include participation in the local chapter of the American Cancer

Society's breast cancer action team and speakers network; volunteering for the Susan G. Komen Foundation New York Affiliate "Race for the Cure" as a speaker/educator at race package pick-up and registration, neighborhood street fairs, corporate luncheons, and health fairs. Serving as a consultant for the state Student Nurses Association and as a career counselor at the National Student Nurses Association annual convention have been energizing experiences as well.

Find something that interests you, perhaps in your area of expertise, with which you are knowledgeable and comfortable. Many worthwhile community organizations would be grateful for your involvement. A word of caution, though: be careful not to overextend yourself so that you fail to keep your commitments to community organizations. Falling back on a commitment will be a major disappointment to the organization and will reflect poorly on you and the college or university you represent. It should go without saying that if you back out of a significant community service commitment without adequate notice, your colleagues on the promotion and tenure review committee will not look favorably on your service obligations.

5. How important is service in the overall scheme of things?

When preparing for tenure, faculty should be aware of the fact that the teaching component, including evaluations (both peer and student); development of new courses and/or programs or curriculum; innovations in teaching; clinical expertise; professional certification; scholarship in the form of research, grant writing, publications, presentations of research, keynote speaking at local, regional, and/or national or international meetings and conferences; serving as a peer reviewer for the scholarly work of others; and national recognition for research expertise carry greater weight than the service contributions. This was validated in Messmer's study of nursing deans' perceptions of faculty performance as related to awarding of tenure. Deans who participated in the study ranked service last, after teaching and research, when deciding to award tenure. In the overall scheme of things, while service is a component of the faculty role, it is often least valued when tenure decisions are made. Faculty who do not participate in service activities, however, are not likely to fare well when promotion and tenure decisions are made.

6. How much time should I devote to service?

Although not stipulated in faculty or policy handbooks, the expectation is at least 4–6 hours per month. Many faculty will attest to providing at least 8–10 hours, with more time expended during summer hours.

7. I am a member of nursing department and college-wide committees, and several task forces. How do I keep from spending all of my time on service activities?

Try to compartmentalize your time. Allocate periods of time that you will spend outside of meetings preparing for upcoming meetings or working on special projects. Sometimes it helps to get started on a committee-related project immediately after the meeting ends, or at the beginning of the next day, while discussion and ideas are fresh in your mind. For example, if you are on a committee that has decided to study a particular issue, and you are the person who volunteered to spearhead the study, you might want to conduct an online literature search to retrieve relevant articles that you will read later. Likewise, if you have agreed to conduct a survey of practices in other colleges or nursing programs, develop the survey as soon as possible after the meeting. The department secretary can begin to develop a database of individuals to whom the survey will be sent. Once the ball is rolling, you can then turn your attention to other activities.

8. Does consulting count as a service activity?

This issue comes up frequently in discussions of faculty service. The operative concept here is *money*. When a faculty member provides consultation to community groups or clinical agencies and/or participates in their continuing education programs *without receiving a consultation fee*, he or she is offering service to that organization. Serving as an "expert witness" *without* requesting a fee is an additional example. Charge a fee for these activities, and you have become an entrepreneur, not a servant!

9. How do I garner support for my ideas as a committee member?

First, "test the waters" by getting to know the climate and dynamics of the group. Change and innovation are often more readily accepted when the participants play an active role in its initiation. Allow participants to address all sides of the issues for the change that you are proposing. You will garner greater support for your idea if it is realistic, appropriate, and economical. Be sure to research all aspects of your proposal and address the positives and negatives as clearly and succinctly as possible.

That done, keep in mind that interpersonal skills and one's character go a long way in garnering support for anything. Colleagues who recognize your open-mindedness and objectivity when considering the ideas of others will be more likely to listen to and support your ideas, if the ideas make sense. If you are respected and trusted by your colleagues, it follows that your ideas will be more readily accepted, or at least heard. However, if you tend to have a short fuse and want things your way, chances are that the committee will be less tolerant of your ideas! The best conceived ideas can go adrift if the person who proposes them is rude and egocentric.

BIBLIOGRAPHY

1. Lynton EA: Making the Case for Professional Service. Forum on Faculty Roles and Rewards. Washington, DC, American Association for Higher Education, 1995.
2. Norbeck JS: Teaching, research, and service: striking the balance in doctoral education. J Prof Nurs 14:197-205, 1998.
3. Park SM: Research, teaching, and service: Why shouldn't women's work count? J Higher Educ 67:46-84, 1996.
4. Schoenfeld AC, Magnan R: Mentor in a Manual: Climbing the Academic Ladder to Tenure, 2nd ed. Madison, WI, Magna, 1994.

8. ACADEMIC ADVISEMENT

Sandra Y. Barnes, PhD, RN

1. What is my role as academic advisor?

The overall faculty role of an academic advisor is designed to assist students in long-range program planning and goal achievement using institutional and community resources. This role includes course selection, considering prerequisites, registration, career counseling, personal growth counseling, and listening/mentoring skills. Advisors need to make sure that the student has the necessary tools for progressing smoothly through the program. These tools include the school catalog, curriculum pattern, admission procedures, including deadlines for submission, course schedules, and other relevant policies and procedures. It is helpful to review handouts with the student to interpret policies and highlight important points. Lastly, advisors must act as advocates and resource persons for information needed by students. This information may include tutoring, counseling, study skills, time management, writing skills, financial aid, health services, or other student support services. Personally facilitating referrals by providing names, phone numbers, directions, and assistance with setting up appointments may be necessary.

2. What should the discussion focus on during the initial advisement meeting?

During the initial advisement meeting, the advisor should define the parameters of the relationship. The initial role entails engaging the student in the advisement relationship by welcoming him/her to the program in person, by letter and/or a phone call. This time should also be used to find out about the student on a personal, as well as an academic level. Advisors should give students their office hours and phone number and request that students speak clearly and slowly when leaving messages on voice mail. It is helpful if advisors inform advisees of the following:

- That you will return phone calls as soon as possible
- How to access the office secretary if there is an urgent matter
- The location of educational aids such as the nursing laboratory, the library, and other areas nursing resources may be located, financial aid office, careers development center, health center, counseling center, etc.
- The rigors of the program, time management, and school policies and procedures. For example, advisees must be clear on policies regarding incomplete grades, repeated courses, withdrawal from classes, and grade point average requirements. Advisees should also be made aware of the appeal process, the disciplinary process, and grievance policies.

3. What is the student's role in the advisement process?

The student's role in the advisement process is usually one of seeking information and having problems resolved. Specifically, students should

- Consult with the advisor on a regular basis
- Study the catalog and other materials to keep abreast of policies and procedures
- Develop short- and long-term career goals
- Clarify information with the advisor

- Use the advisor as a consultant for academic and nonacademic issues
- Be prompt for appointments, bringing all necessary working documents and questions
- Call to reschedule appointments if necessary
- Be honest in discussions with the advisor
- Seek out the advisor in a timely fashion
- Assume a fair share of developing an alliance with the advisor.

Students should also be cautioned against seeking out different faculty members for assistance, when possible, to maintain consistency and avoid errors in advisement.

4. How often should I meet with my advisees?

Faculty should meet with advisees as often as necessary. However, a meeting once or twice a semester should suffice for most students. A mid-term meeting helps to see how things are progressing and to identify student problems at an early stage. Early assessment and intervention can help the student to be successful if there are problems. This meeting should also be used to remind the student about an end-of-semester meeting that is designed to help prepare the student for early registration and other time lines that must be met for the next semester.

5. How much time should I allow for advisement?

Time allotted for advisement should vary according to the individual needs of the student. A well-organized, prepared student may require only 5–10 minutes of contact, whereas a student with multiple problems, questions, and concerns may require 15–30 minutes or more. Possible time required should be estimated at the time the appointment is made.

6. What kind of records should advisors keep?

Advisors should keep accurate records in the department related to students' progress toward graduation. Records should also include personal notes from dated meetings, transcripts, grade reports, checklists of departmental requirements, reasons students drop or withdraw from school, copies of letters of recommendation, as well as other pertinent academic information.

7. What if the student's parents request a meeting with me?

If parents request a meeting, it is fine to meet as long as the student is aware of the request and in attendance at the same meeting. This is a wonderful way to involve the family in a supportive role, as well as to learn more about the individual needs of the student. As many nursing students are now older adult learners, a spouse may request a conference. However, the same rules apply. If the student consents to the request and is in attendance at the same meeting, we can try to form an alliance to meet the goals of the student.

8. Is there any difference in advising undergraduate and graduate students?

There is little difference in advising undergraduate and graduate students today because many are adult learners who tend to be more self-directed and take a more active role in seeking out information and being aware of program requirements. Some students may be traditional students, entering college straight from high school, and still be quite adept at taking charge of their educational processes when we assume that they may need more guidance. Both assumptions may not always hold true, hence the need for individualized advisement with all students. The major difference in advising undergraduates and graduate students would possibly entail assisting a graduate student with thesis or research projects.

9.   Is there any difference in advising transfer and RN completion students compared to generic students?

The major difference in advising transfer and RN completion students is to ensure clear articulation, in contrast to generic students, who present with a high school or general education degree. Students must understand exactly what course transfer credit they will receive, what is nontransferable, and which courses need to be repeated. Transfer students may also find information on the College Level Examination Program (CLEP) useful. RNs need to know if there are requirements for demonstrating clinical skills, and if there is any flexibility in selecting clinical sites and types of clinical experiences. Once this is done, transfer students need to understand exactly how long it will take to complete the program, taking into account course sequencing and scheduling. Differences in school policies and procedures also need to be clearly explained to transfer students. Lastly, RN completion students may need more peer support and encouragement to proceed methodically to ensure success as they frequently have family, employment, and other responsibilities. The fable of the tortoise and the hare works well here to illustrate the point that sometimes it is necessary to go more slowly to win the race.

10.   Are there other students with special needs?

Yes. Students with disabilities may require additional advisement and accommodations to facilitate successful outcomes. If students present disabilities that they have not declared, they should be sent to the Office of Students with Disabilities to assist them with special learning needs and support groups. Other students who may require additional services would include students with alcohol and substance abuse problems, mental health problems, date rape, and domestic violence.

11.   What should I do if I make an error in advisement?

If an advisor makes an error in advisement, genuinely apologize to the student and then see if and how any damage can be minimized. The error should then be used as a learning process to avoid future errors. One of the main ways to avoid such errors is to keep abreast of policy and programmatic changes not only in the department, but in the school at large. Students should be considerate of human error and respectful of the advisor's role as a helping agent.

12.   What information can I include in a letter of reference for my advisees if I know them only in the advisor/advisee capacity?

An advisor can always include the student's overall grade point average in a reference letter, any classes they have had that might be related to the position for which they are applying, the length of time they have known the advisee, participation and roles in student organizations, volunteer services, and some of the personal/professional characteristics they have noted about the advisee.

13.   What should I do if an academically weak advisee asks me to write a letter of reference?

There are several ways to handle this situation. The first is to refuse to write the letter and be honest in explaining why to the student. If it is anticipated that a weak advisee might ask for a letter of reference in the future, he or she can be forewarned that you will not be able to write a reference letter. Another way to handle this situation is to note the student's initial difficulty with the program, then note that the student has demonstrated marked improvement personally and professionally in his/her ability to achieve goals. Also, the positive characteristics that would be job assets can be pointed out. Lastly, a letter could be written pointing out only the positive work-related characteristics if you have firsthand knowledge of the student's performance in a work-related role such as teaching assistant, research assistant, or student aide.

14. What are my legal responsibilities regarding the advisement process?

Legally, faculty advisors should be familiar with several documents to assist special students, avoid discrimination, and maximize the student's educational experience. Faculty should be familiar with the Family Education Rights and Privacy Act (FERPA), also known as the Buckley Amendment. This Act speaks to the rights of students to access their educational records and files, as well as maintaining confidentiality of the records. Faculty should also be aware of the fourteenth constitutional amendment, which addresses equal rights of citizenship and thus ensures due process for students. The first amendment ensures freedom of speech and freedom of religious expression. Laws regarding special students and the prevention of discrimination based upon disability include the Rehabilitation Act of 1973 and the American Disabilities Act of 1990. The Education Amendments of 1972 prohibit sexual discrimination in educational practices. The Civil Rights Acts of 1871, 1875, 1957 and 1960 also address discrimination and violation of one's civil rights. When in doubt about the rights of students, the legal department of the campus should be consulted. Additionally, school policies and procedures should be respected, accessible to students, and consistent with federal and state laws.

BIBLIOGRAPHY

1. Cullen P et al: An issue of conflicting rights: Nursing student charged with drug trafficking. J Prof Nurs 13:186-192, 1997.
2. Kearney RT: Academic advisement and the RN-to-BSN student. J Cont Educ Nurs 25:11-16, 1994.
3. Maheady DC: Jumping through hoops, walking on eggshells: The experiences of nursing students with disabilities. J Nurs Educ 38:162-170, 1999.
4. NACADA Statement of Core Values of Academic Advising. National Academic Advisors Association J 15:5-7, 1995.
5. Parkes BS, et al: Academic support program for high-risk students. J Nurs Educ 35: 331-333, 1996.
6. Roberts VW et al: Coping with declining resources and escalating enrollments: An alternative advisement strategy. J Nurs Educ 33: 376-377, 1994.
7. Sherrod RA, Harrison L: Evaluation of a comprehensive advisement program designed to enhance student retention. Nurse Educator 19:29-33, 1994.
8. Schultz ED: Academic advising from a nursing theory perspective. Nurse Educator 23:22-25, 1998.
9. Trent BA: Student perceptions of academic advising in an RN-to-BSN program. J Cont Educ Nurs 28:276-283, 1997.

III. Negotiating the System

9. FACULTY WORKLOAD

Dolores A. Bower, PhD, RN, and Vicki Smith, MSN, RN

1. What is faculty workload?

Faculty workload is defined as the time spent on all professionally appropriate activities, directly or indirectly related to teaching, research, or service. Faculty workload includes three components: teaching, scholarly activities, and service. Service may be further defined as internal (department, college, or university) or external (professional or community activities). Faculty load is used synonymously with faculty workload, but is not to be confused with teaching load.[1]

2. How does faculty workload differ from teaching load?

Faculty workload is the *sum* of its components, whereas teaching is only one component of workload. Because teaching tends to dominate the work of a faculty member and can be relatively easy to compute, it tends to become the "baseline" for the work expectations of a faculty member.

3. What constitutes "teaching" load?

Teaching load refers to the amount of time the teacher/instructor is engaged in the teaching/learning process with a number of students. Teaching load can refer to clinical, classroom, or laboratory instruction. The credit that an instructor receives for teaching depends on the setting and number of students involved in the teaching activity. Many institutions also consider academic advisement as part of the teaching component.

4. Does the typical faculty workload differ between public and private institutions?

The literature indicates that private institutions tend to emphasize teaching and service, whereas public agencies identify research and scholarship as a priority.[1] The emphasis may change from year to year, depending on select activities such as program accreditation, monetary grants, or goals of the nursing unit or university.

5. How is workload expressed?

Workload can be expressed in hours per week, hours per semester, or duties per semester.

6. How do you calculate faculty workload?

Historically there are several methods to calculate faculty workload; however, none has been totally satisfactory. Faculty workload may be defined and computed in terms of assigned credit hours, student credit hours per full-time equivalent, contact hours, student/faculty ratio, and workload formulas. Workload studies indicate that contact hours tend to reflect the total hours devoted to a course, including preparation, grading and other

61

activities. For example, if a faculty assignment included teaching 12 course credits, the calculation would be as follows:

$$12 \ (credit \ hours) \ x \ 15 \ (weeks \ per \ semester) = 180 \ contact \ hours \ per \ semester$$

Therefore, the faculty member would have to teach four 3-credit hour courses, each totaling 45 contact hours, in order to reach the teaching load requirement. In an early study conducted by Coudret,[3] nursing faculty preferred a formula method of calculating workload because it allowed flexibility within the department and was based on need, interest, and ability rather than a strict adherence to a uniform workload assignment.

7. What factors affect faculty workload?

One of the most frequently reported factors affecting faculty workload is that different amounts of time are required for adequate preparation and effective teaching of different subjects. The instructional setting is also a major factor affecting workload of nursing faculty. The amount of time devoted to preparation and instructional delivery can vary greatly between a classroom, campus laboratory, or clinical site. It takes much longer to prepare new material than it does to update previously taught material, one variable that is usually not factored in workload calculations. Class size, graduate versus undergraduate students, and subject matter may also affect the amount of time required for effective teaching. Other factors that may affect workload include the type of institution in which the faculty member works and university mission.

8. What effect does clinical instruction have on total workload?

The most obvious difference between clinical and classroom instruction is the structure of the setting. Clinical teaching occurs in a hospital, clinic, community agency, or other practice setting. Clinical settings can usually accommodate no more than 8-10 students (fewer in high-acuity settings) during one time period and, therefore, limits the student-to-instructor ratio. Because of this, many universities decrease the credit given to the instructor for the time spent with the student. It is this ratio that often drives the formula of a 1:2 ratio of contact hour/credit to clock hours, rather than 1:1 ratio that is the standard contact credit given to a classroom course. In other words, the clinical instructor must teach 6 hours of face-to-face contact with the student in clinical settings to receive 3 contact hours of credit toward his or her workload. Using the American Association of University Professors' guide of 12 weekly contact hours, 24–36 clock hours per week would be spent on teaching activities (teaching class, preparation time, and evaluation of learning). The rest of the time would be spent on service and scholarly activity. When clinical instruction is part of workload, the number of clock hours increases in order to obtain the required number or contact hours. Therefore, the amount of time the instructor can devote to service and scholarly activities decreases.

9. What clinical workload ratio is desirable and why?

The most desirable workload is one that allows the faculty to do scholarly and service activities. As the number of hours spent teaching clinical courses increases, the amount of time remaining for other activities decreases. Therefore, the most desirable teaching ratio is one that uses 1:1 (clock hour to credit).

10. How much time does a faculty member have left after teaching responsibilities to spend on scholarly and service activities?

Time spent on nonteaching activities depends on the workload ratio, especially when teaching in clinical and the classroom. Schuster and colleagues surveyed 22 baccalaureate programs and discovered that nursing faculty who taught clinical courses with 0.5:1 to

0.25:1 workload credit for face-to-face contact hour ratios needed to work between 8 and 24 hours more in face-to-face teaching compared to colleagues teaching lecture courses. Schuster and colleagues concluded that these teachers had less time to meet scholarship and service requirements of their faculty workload.

11. Should faculty practice affect contract workload?

Absolutely, especially if maintaining one's practice is a faculty expectation. Many institutions consider practice as a type of scholarship. The conclusion can be made that a faculty member who is engaged in practice is current and competent in his or her specialty, as well as in teaching.

12. How does workload affect tenure requirements?

Workload unmistakably affects the tenure process. All components of workload must be balanced and taken into account when readying oneself for tenure. If the instructor has clinical teaching responsibilities, the time left for scholarly activity depends on how the contact hours are calculated in that particular institution.

13. How do nursing faculty loads compare to other disciplines in the university?

Nursing faculty loads are often not the same as other academic disciplines. Since clinical contact hours are often not calculated in the same way as classroom contact hours, the credits computed for nursing faculty will ultimately increase the clock hours working. Schuster noted that nursing faculty may not have an equal opportunity to compete for promotion and tenure with other faculty who teach lecture courses within the university setting. Studies reported in the nursing literature raise concerns about faculty expectations in workload and potential barriers to rewards. If nursing faculty have excessive teaching responsibilities, they will not be able to reach the research and scholarship expectations that usually lead to promotion and tenure.

14. What do studies of faculty workload tell us?

Despite some standard guides, there is great variance in the way that faculty spend their time. There is variance within departments, between colleges within the university, and among universities. Some disciplines, such as nursing, have special challenges because of the instructional methods used.

BIBLIOGRAPHY

1. Bower DA: Faculty Workload in Two Selected Baccalaureate Schools of Nursing. Unpublished dissertation Kent, OH, Kent State University, 1983.
2. Boyer E: Scholarship Reconsidered: Priorities of the Professoriate. Princeton, The Carnegie Foundation for the Advancement of Teaching, 1990.
3. Coudret NA: Determining faculty workload. Nurse Educator 6:38-41, 1981.
4. Fong CM: A longitudinal study of the relationships between overload, social support, and burnout among nursing educators. J Nurs Educ 32:24-29, 1993.
5. Oermann MH: Work-related stress of clinical nursing faculty. J Nurs Educ 37:302-304, 1998.
6. Ruby J: Baccalaureate nurse educators' workload and productivity: ascription of values and the challenges of evaluation. J NY State Nurses Assoc 29:18-22, 1998.
7. Schuster P, Fitzgerald DC, McCarthy PA, McDougal, D: Workload issues in clinical nursing education. J Prof Nurs 13:154-159, 1997.

10. FACULTY EVALUATION

Dolores A. Bower, PhD, RN, and Ann H. Venuto, MS, RN

1. What does faculty evaluation mean?

In its broadest sense, the term faculty evaluation refers to the appraisal of a faculty member's work, which includes teaching, research, scholarship, and service. Evaluation data usually contribute to decisions about hiring, retention, reappointment, promotion, and tenure. The term faculty evaluation is frequently used interchangeably with teaching evaluations. This chapter will focus on issues related to evaluation of faculty teaching.

2. Who evaluates faculty teaching?

Many people can evaluate the teaching of a faculty member. They include administrators, peers, alumni, and students. Depending on the type of instruction, other stakeholders may be appropriate, such as practitioners in health care agencies, and the public. Self-evaluations are also considered appropriate when used in conjunction with other sources. Though student ratings are most commonly used, most authorities agree that multiple sources of data are essential to obtaining an accurate profile of teaching effectiveness.[4]

3. How do you measure effective classroom teaching?

The first task is to determine what is effective classroom teaching. The areas that should be assessed include *content expertise, delivery skills,* and an *aptitude for instructional design*. Though standard instruments or questionnaires are available and may be adapted to one's own program, faculty do need to determine what areas will be evaluated, what sources of data are appropriate, when will data be collected, and, finally, what kind of measure will be used.

Validity and reliability of any measure must be considered. When students are the source of feedback, give a priority to brevity and clarity. A rating scale with space to add comments is typically used.

4. Are there any guidelines for determining the type and number of data sources for evaluating teaching?

The guidelines are simple and logical. First, decide on your definition of effective teaching. Second, identify sources of evaluation data that will provide the best information about teaching effectiveness. The following table provides an example of best sources to assess particular aspects of teaching:

ASPECT OF TEACHING	DATA SOURCES
Subject mastery	Self, peer
Course content and design	Self, peer, student, supervisor
Classroom delivery	Self, peer, student, supervisor

Self-evaluations may take the form of a portfolio that is gaining in use and popularity.

5. How can effective clinical teaching be measured?

Everyone would agree that clinical instruction is very important in a nursing program, yet how can we be sure that all clinical instruction is effective? The first step, as with classroom instruction, is to decide what behaviors indicate effective clinical teaching. The next step is to develop a matrix for sources of data. The following table provides an example:

DOMAINS OF CLINICAL TEACHING	DATA SOURCES
Clinical competence	Self, nurse manager, clients
Organization of experiences	Self, nurse manager, students
Interpersonal skills	Nurse manager, students, clients

Numerous studies in the nursing literature identify effective clinical teaching behaviors. Defining the relationship between student and teacher at different levels in the program seems to be an important step. Once identified, an instrument, such as the rating scale developed by Fong and McCauley,[7] can be used. The Clinical Teaching Evaluation (CTE) tool assesses the instructor's skill in relating underlying theory to clinical practice situations. *Are there reliability and validity data available? Does the instrument assess the domains of clinical teaching identified in the table?*

6. Should student feedback be considered a valid indicator of faculty teaching performance?

Yes, when providing data about a dimension of teaching that students are qualified to evaluate. Student ratings are best used in measuring aspects of teaching that affect students, such as: clarity of delivery, availability of the instructor, and willingness to answer questions.

Validity of student evaluation is increased when anonymity is guaranteed. If students believe that they can be identified, they will be reluctant to share their honest feelings. It is much harder to assure anonymity and confidentiality in small groups. By taking the following steps, the instructor can increase the validity of student feedback:

- No student names or other identifiers on evaluation forms
- Instructor leaves room while students complete the ratings
- Instructor does not handle surveys until summarized
- Surveys should not be reviewed before grades are computed to avoid faculty bias or the perception by students that surveys impact grading

7. What about peer evaluations of teaching effectiveness?

Although it can also pose some inherent difficulties, a peer review system can stimulate improvement in teaching effectiveness. Some critics believe that a close colleague will rarely give anything but an excellent review during a classroom observation. On the other hand, some faculty regard evaluation by peers as more meaningful than student feedback because colleagues have broader perspectives and a greater familiarity with course and program objectives.

In order to achieve more objectivity, evaluation criteria must be explicit, understood by all faculty, and periodically reviewed. Materials such as syllabi, course objectives, exam questions, and handouts can be collected for the reviewer. In addition to standardized tools, some advocate the use of faculty reviewers from outside the nursing department, although most schools rely on the use of academic supervisors and peers from within the nursing department. Ideally, more than one or two observations are necessary to evaluate teaching effectiveness, although Crawford[6] reported that less than half of the schools of nursing surveyed used more than one observation.

8. How are evaluation data used?

Evaluation data may be formative or summative. The same measure can be used to collect data for either purpose. Therefore it is important that the purpose is clear prior to developing instruments or collecting data.

9. What is the difference between formative and summative evaluation?

Formative evaluations are used to support faculty growth, development, and self-improvement, whereas summative evaluation enables administration to make decisions about retention, promotion, and tenure.

Faculty need to be aware of the way in which the data will be used and to distinguish between the two types of evaluation. When faculty are committed to professional growth and development, they will welcome the honest critical feedback that students and peers can offer through a formative evaluation process.

10. Can faculty evaluations be both formative and summative?

Yes, though there is much disagreement about whether a faculty evaluation program can be both formative and summative and still be effective. One view insists that appraisals of faculty to stimulate improvement must remain distinct from those whose purpose is promotion and retention. Because no known models exist to guarantee the separation, the opposing view gains strength. It promotes the incorporation of both purposes in a single faculty evaluation system. On the surface, faculty and administrators may agree that improving teaching effectiveness is the primary purpose of faculty evaluation; however, their perceptions may be quite different as to whether or not that purpose is accomplished. That difference in perception is likely to inhibit the success of a faculty evaluation system that attempts to combine formative and summative aspects.

Faculty fears about the evaluation process are commonplace when formative and summative aspects are combined in the same process. Such a system can generate a climate of mistrust when data reportedly used for self-improvement may all too easily become data used for personnel decision-making by administration.

11. What is a teaching portfolio?

A teaching portfolio is a teacher-developed collection of documents that support teaching activities. It may include certificates, degrees, licenses, letters of support from colleagues, syllabi, handouts, peer evaluations, summary of student evaluations, graded assignments, and a philosophy of teaching.

12. What makes a successful faculty evaluation program?

A faculty evaluation program should be a systematic process, developed in a climate of trust, and mutually agreed upon by faculty and the institution. It should be comprehensive and employ a variety of objective measures and use multiple sources. It should be both formative and summative, with emphasis on faculty growth and development. The formative evaluation has the potential for going beyond simple feedback about performance to rewarding faculty members with an experience of affirmation and an extensive blueprint for professional growth. This type of milieu creates a win-win situation for all the players: the institution, which gains more satisfied, energized and dedicated faculty, and the students, who receive high-quality educational programs.

13. What are the latest trends in faculty evaluations?

Barber et al.[2] described the application to a user-friendly, online interactive evaluation program that uses code names for the students to assure anonymity. ALT, an alternative newspaper in Buffalo, NY, has initiated a website to collect data on professors at four colleges in the community. The student wishing to share observations writes a comment on the course, specifically focusing on the teaching skills of the instructor. Professors may find this trend alarming, since anyone who has access to the Internet can acquire this information.

Total quality management (TQM) or continuous quality management (CQM) has been enthusiastically adopted at numerous community colleges to evaluate clerical and staff performance. There have been a number of innovative programs across the county utilizing TQM. This represents a paradigm shift in faculty evaluation from a hierarchical to a collegial process. Nurses may be more familiar with TQM principles than other college educators because these principles are "old news" in health care institutions.

BIBLIOGRAPHY

1. Andrews H: TQM and Faculty Evaluation: Ever the Twain Shall Meet? ERIC Digest, April 1997.
2. Barber K, Wyatt K, Gerbasi F: On-line interactive evaluation in course and clinical instruction. Nurse Educator 24: 37-40, 1999.
3. Bower DA, Linc L, Denega D: Evaluation Instruments in Nursing. New York, National League for Nursing, 1988.
4. Cashin WE: Student Ratings of Teaching: Recommendation for Use. IDEA Paper No. 22. Manhattan, KS, Kansas State University, Center for Faculty Evaluation and Development, 1990.
5. Cashin WE: Student Ratings of Teaching: The Research Revisited, IDEA paper No.32. Manhattan, KS, Kansas State University, Manhattan Center for Faculty Evaluation and Development in Higher Education, 1995.
6. Crawford LH: Evaluation of nursing faculty through observation. J Nurs Educ 37: 289-94, 1998.
7. Fong CM, McCauley GT: Measuring the nursing, teaching and interpersonal effectiveness of clinical instructors. J Nurs Educ 32:325-8, 1993.
8. Koon J, Murray HG: Using multiple outcomes to validate student ratings of overall teacher effectiveness. J Higher Educ 66:61-81, 1995.
9. Rifkin T: The Status and Scope of Faculty Evaluation. ERIC Digest, Los Angeles, CA, ERIC Clearinghouse for Community Colleges, June 1995.

11. MENTORING NEW FACULTY

Anita L. Throwe, MS, RN, CS, *and Sandra B. Weatherford*, MSN, RN, FNP, CEN

1. What is mentoring?

Mentoring is a process by which an experienced faculty member befriends and guides a new faculty member in his or her career development. The mentor shares experiences, knowledge, and wisdom with the mentee, who is learning how to become an expert in a chosen career or who is making a career change from clinical practice to the academic setting. The mentoring process can help a neophyte faculty member to more quickly learn the "game plan" of the institution. Thus, mentoring is a catalytic process that guides and speeds up the role socialization process for a new faculty member. Current evidence exists that mentoring relationships do work in the socialization of new faculty and should be supported.

The Mentoring Connection
Facilitating Role Acquisition

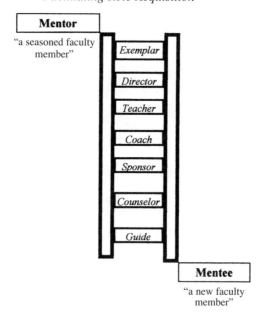

Mentor
"a seasoned faculty member"

Exemplar

Director

Teacher

Coach

Sponsor

Counselor

Guide

Mentee
"a new faculty member"

2. How does a mentor differ from a preceptor, apprentice, or role model?

Sometimes the mentor is seen as a role model, preceptor, or master in a master-apprentice relationship, but the role is more than that. Some apprenticeships are void of interpersonal involvement and function solely to enable learning the craft. Role models can be just that—someone to emulate and admire sometimes from afar or with minimal contact. Preceptors are usually assigned by the organization to provide time-limited assistance for a new employee to learn the policy, procedures, job description, expectations, and requirements of the position. The focus in the assigned (preceptor) relationship is on task accomplishment and proficiency during an orientation period, and is usually devoid of any long-term commitment aimed at encouraging personal and professional growth. Preceptor/neophyte relationships can develop into mentor/mentee relationships; however, most do not.

The mentor relationship is voluntary for both parties and is built on mutual respect and the potential development of the mentee. Mentors share time, experience, and expertise; in turn, mentors should be stimulated by the mentee's ideas and challenged to read and think more deeply. Both individual and professional growth are rewards that stem from the relationship.

3. What is the advantage for a new faculty member in having a mentor?

One can get along, and even succeed, without a mentor. However, the mentorship experience is advantageous for the mentee (the new faculty member), the mentor (the experienced faculty member), the profession, and the academic environment, for all gain from such a relationship. The mentee, while "under the wing" of the mentor, can expect accelerated role development, and psychological and professional support. This is important, especially for female professionals, as women generally are not accustomed to having unselfish sponsorship. Some research cites greater personal satisfaction, increased self-confidence, and enhanced self-esteem as an advantage of a mentor connection.

4. What is in it for the mentor?

The benefits of becoming a mentor are often intangible and difficult to describe. However, some of the "gains" for the mentor include:

- The opportunity to provide advice or consultation, through the mentee's network, to other novice faculty, which enables the mentor to develop additional collegial relationships that otherwise might not have developed.
- A new and different perspective on current issues and trends, especially important in academia where the goal is to foster critical thinking and inquiry.
- The opportunity to make significant contributions to society and to fulfill one's personal need to affect the future of one's chosen profession by helping to cultivate and guide the next generation of faculty.

5. What is the mentee's responsibility to the mentor?

First and foremost, the mentee should be familiar with the published guidelines for rank expectation (job description and the triad components of teaching, research, and service). Seeking guidance from, and coaching by, the selected mentor, then, provides a good starting point for developing the mentoring process.

Once the relationship is underway, the mentee's responsibilities to the mentor include:
- Display an eagerness to learn the faculty role components.
- Demonstrate a commitment toward excellence in fulfilling the faculty role components.
- Participate as a "partner" and keep all commitments.
- Seek constructive feedback and, when appropriate, modify behaviors.
- Maintain open dialogue and participate in extensive discussions regarding faculty role development.
- Trust that the mentor's plan will facilitate one's role development goal.
- Be supportive, flexible, and open to change.
- Initiate help offers at critical times during the semester (midterm, end of course, and at grant deadlines) to provide the mentor with assistance by performing selected tasks (monitoring examinations, test proofing, reference letter writing, etc.).
- BE LOYAL TO YOUR MENTOR!

- Avoid becoming overly dependent on the mentor by diminishing the number of interactions seeking guidance and direction. This can be accomplished by:
  - enhancing one's problem solving abilities
  - identifying choices and options
  - seeking validation of choices
  - acting on one's choices
  - evaluating one's choices and outcomes

6. How should I select a mentor?

Finding a mentor can be a challenge. When selecting a mentor, recognize the characteristics that make one an effective mentor. Seek a mentor who is, generally, an older, wiser, more
experienced member of the nursing professoriate, who has earned the respect of colleagues, and
who is considered to be an expert. Additionally, your potential mentor should set high standards
for herself or himself, have demonstrated a measure of superior achievement, and show an
interest in your career development. Qualities to look for in a potential mentor include:
- Good communication skills
- Sensitivity to the needs of others
- The ability to counsel
- An understanding of power and its utilization
- A willingness to share
- Good decision-making abilities
- Trustworthiness
- The ability to encourage excellence in others

7. What should I do if the chemistry just is not right between my mentor and me?

In a preceptor relationship that is time limited, one can "grin and bear" the relationship or
ask to be reassigned to another preceptor. However, in a mentor-mentee relationship, which is
usually initiated by the mentee, then you will need to do some soul searching to analyze what
has gone wrong. In the process, try to re-engage the former level of trust to continue the relationship, if that is your desired outcome. With analysis comes insight into one's behavior and,
then, purposeful actions can be taken with the present relationship and/or applied to future collegial relationships. It is important to remember that you have control only over your behavior
and, therefore, cannot force the intensity of the relationship for the other person. A mentor-
mentee relationship is like all personal relationships that have both intense and less intense periods. The less intense period is necessary to allow mentee and mentor time for self and time to
focus on other work-related activities before reconnecting, where the focus will, again, be on
helping the mentee with career development. If the relationship has become oppressive to you,
and you do not want to continue it, then figure out a way to disengage from the relationship
intensity without closing the door with a final slam!

**8. Can new faculty assume that the institution will assign a mentor to aid in the social-
ization process?**

No. Often, a new inexperienced nursing faculty member is assigned to teach either as a
member of a course team or under the direction of a course coordinator. All new faculty can
expect to undergo faculty orientation to become familiar with college or university policies
and procedures and be given faculty and student handbooks for reference. Very few institutions have implemented a formal mentoring connection. While this connection may be
encouraged, most often it is individually sought rather than set in an organized fashion.
Deans and directors would do well to sanction the mentor connection and provide time and
incentives for its development. Mentoring is an excellent strategy to assist new faculty with

role enactment and to increase job satisfaction in a very competitive academic environment.

Pearl: Advice to the newly employed faculty member: Seek your own mentor and do not expect administration to "issue" a mentor.

9. Are there any disadvantages to participating in a mentor-mentee relationship?

If you choose to participate in a mentoring relationship, then anticipate that the advantages will far outweigh the disadvantages. However, your mentor-mentee relationship might experience one or more of the following disadvantages:

- *Time and energy consuming.* Mentoring requires time and energy as well as an element of risk-taking behavior.
- *No guarantees of success.* There are no guarantees that the time and energy spent by your mentor will result in your becoming a successful, fully socialized faculty colleague. Learning (role-acquisition) is your responsibility! Moreover, the time factor for goal achievement will vary for each individual.
- *Emotional intensity.* The mentoring relationship can be emotionally intense, since the mentor has accepted responsibility for guiding and protecting the mentee. Sometimes this results in envy by other nurse faculty colleagues who may view the mentoring connection as a power coalition. However, this is not the goal of a mentoring relationship.

10. What should I do if I don't agree with my mentor's advice?

You, the mentee, are in the position to either accept or reject the guidance and direction being offered by your mentor. Your mentor should be prepared to accept your decision. Sometimes an overzealous mentor, in his or her eagerness to help the mentee achieve identified professional goals, will become oppressive and controlling, and foster over-dependency. A good mentor will recognize the dependency and facilitate the mentee's movement toward independence. So, choose wisely when selecting a mentor.

11. How long should a mentoring relationship exist?

The relationship has no definite time limits and individually varies with each dyad. One way of conceptualizing the relationship is to view it in light of Maslow's human needs model. Using this model as a framework, the relationship should begin at the security stage and progress until the mentee's personal and professional actualization have been achieved. This should be evident when the mentee is confident in fulfilling all components of the faculty role. For many faculty, the mentoring connection is sustained throughout one's entire career. Sometimes this life-long relationship varies in intensity. The relationship may even wane, but if it has been an effective relationship, it should easily be rekindled to allow for periodic validation of choices, challenges, and opportunities by the mentee or the mentor.

12. What is the ultimate goal of a mentor-mentee relationship?

The goal of the mentoring relationship is to provide guidance, support, inspiration, challenge, and protection to a "younger," less experienced faculty member as he or she works toward establishing himself or herself as a fully socialized contributor to the profession. It further serves to provide the mentor with an opportunity to repay the benefits he or she has previously derived from the profession. The mentor connection can be valuable to the profession, as it grooms future leaders and humanizes the sometimes seemingly inhumane world of academe. The ultimate goal of the mentoring relationship, however, is to launch the mentee when self-reliance has occurred. Termination of the mentoring relationship may, then, evolve into a friendship or a collegial relationship.

The Beginning Stages of the Mentoring Affiliation

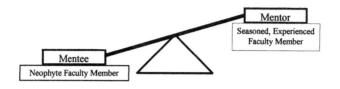

Ultimate Goal of a Mentor Connection

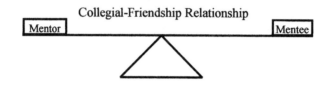

13. Why are nursing faculty somewhat reluctant to aid in the socialization process for new faculty?

Primarily because most colleges and universities do not support mentoring relationships in a formal, recognizable way (release time, merit, advancement, and tenure) to those faculty who willingly participate in this developmental process.

14. As a new faculty researcher, should I expect to have more than one research mentor?

Early in the research experience it is wise to seek a mentor to help advance your research abilities. Later, as you advance in the nurse–scientist role, it is important to expand from a dyad mentor relationship to interacting with a team of mentors. Three distinct stages are noted, along with the corresponding benefits for a research faculty member.

- *Stage 1: Basic doctoral experiences.* Through anecdotal case observation by the authors, it is noted that mentoring is the process that is most critical to successful completion of doctoral program requirements and for opening the door to a successful scientific career. This interactive process serves both the mentee and mentor in their scientific career advancement.
- *Stage 2: Postdoctoral experiences.* The guidance, expertise, and research focus of a senior mentor are usually considered the major criteria for selecting a postdoctoral study focus and site.
- *Stage 3: One mentor vs. a team of mentors.* Generally, as one advances in the nurse scientist role, it is better to consider branching from a single mentor to a team of mentors (in one's scientific area of inquiry) with connections to a long-term research program. Working with nurse colleagues and colleagues from other disciplines helps one move toward investigator status. It is at this point that the mentee can expect to be the mentor for other less experienced nurse scientists.

15. From the perspective of the mentee, what are the values of participating in a mentor/mentee relationship?

While there are many values cited in the literature, those referred to most often include:

- Discussing strategies to handle professional situations (work- and student-related)
- Providing new opportunities for participation in professional activities (poster presentations, abstract writing, grant writing, manuscript preparation, test construction and analysis, research participation, and development of course syllabi)
- Providing professional advice regarding academic promotion and tenure (re-negotiating contracts; workload; and time management for research, service, and teaching role expectations)
- Observing the mentor in his or her role performance in difficult situations in the academic role (classroom, committees, student advisement and counseling, clinical teaching, and conducting research)
- Gaining access to the mentor's network and being skillfully guided along one's career path (empowering and competency-building qualities)
- Being encouraged in one's role development
- Having another see potential in us that we are frequently unaware of (nudging us to reach beyond our comfort zone, sometimes before we think we are ready)

BIBLIOGRAPHY

1. Brown HN: Mentoring new faculty. Nurse Educator 24:48-51, 1999.
2. Cunningham S: The nature of workplace mentoring relationships among faculty members in Christian higher education. J Higher Educ 70:441-3, 1999.
3. Kavoosi M, Elman N, Mauch J: Faculty mentoring and administrative support in schools of nursing. J Nurs Educ 34:19-26, 1995.
4. Magnussen L: Ensuring success: The faculty development plan. Nurse Educator 22:30-3, 1997.
5. Nugent KE, Bradshaw MJ, Kito N: Teacher self-efficacy in new nurse educators. J Prof Nurs 15:229-37, 1999.
6. Sands RG, Parson L, Duane J: Faculty mentoring faculty in a public university. J Higher Educ 62: 174-193, 1991.
7. Triolo PK, Pozehl B, Mahaffey T: Development of leadership within the university and beyond: Challenges to faculty and their development. J Prof Nurs 13: 149-53, 1997.
8. Van Velsor E, Hughes MW: Gender Differences in the Development of Managers: How Women Managers Learn from Experience. Greensboro, NC, Center for Creative Leadership, 1990.

12. PREPARING FOR TENURE

Anne Manton, PhD, RN, CEN

1. What is tenure?

General dictionary definitions of tenure refer to a term of holding something, such as an office or a position, or a status granted after a trial position. Tenure in the academic setting has come to mean a protected status, granted after a probationary period, in which certain protections are guaranteed. Included among those protections is continuation of the academic appointment until retirement, with exception for cause or other well-defined circumstances.

2. What is the purpose of tenure?

Tenure has several purposes. Foremost among those purposes is the ensuring of academic freedom. Academic freedom is believed to be essential to free expression, professional autonomy and integrity, and the ability of faculty to contribute to the search for truth through research. Another purpose of tenure is to increase the attractiveness of higher education as a career choice.

3. How did the tenure system come about in higher education?

Principles for tenure were originally put forth in 1925; however, these statements were reiterated and put forth again in 1940 as the "Statement of Principles on Academic Freedom and Tenure." These statements carried the endorsement of both the American Association of University Professors (AAUP) and the Association of American Colleges (AAC). These statements are most commonly referred to when issues of tenure are being discussed. While tenure had existed prior to the issuance of these statements, following their release, tenure became more and more the norm in institutions of higher education.

Interpretative statements, formulated by a joint committee of AAUP and AAC, were added to the guidelines in 1970 as a means of refining the original statement. In 1990 further modifications were made in the language of the statements, including changes made to remove gender-specific language.

4. What are the benefits of tenure to me as an individual?

As stated in the 1940 principles and the 1970 interpretive statements, tenure provides the individual faculty member with the freedom in teaching and research necessary to provide students and the larger society the opportunity to seek and learn the truth without fear of reprisals or recriminations. It supports academic freedom and autonomy, and also provides a degree of economic security.

5. Do all colleges and universities have a tenure system?

Not all colleges and universities have tenure systems, although most do. Even if the college or university does have a tenure system, not all faculty positions are considered tenure track positions. An increasingly controversial issue is the number of faculty hired for "nontenure track" positions. Typically, nontenure track positions are limited term positions (for example, a 1-year appointment), part-time positions, and positions in which the faculty member does not have an earned doctorate. In nursing, many nontenure track positions are filled by clinical faculty.

In some institutions, a model is used in which all faculty members are hired for a specified period of time (for example, 3 years). During this time they must apply for reappointment for the next 3-year cycle. It is important for faculty, upon hire, to have this aspect of the position clearly stated in the contract.

6. When is tenure usually granted?

In most colleges and universities, faculty can apply for tenure after a standard probationary period. Application for tenure is most often made during the sixth year of employment at a rank of instructor or higher. Recommendations of the 1940 Statement of Principles on Academic Freedom and tenure state that "the probationary period should not exceed seven years, including within this period service in all institutions of higher education." This means that faculty who have taught elsewhere, holding the rank of instructor or higher, should receive "credit" for that experience, thus shortening the probationary period at the institution where tenure is being sought.

7. What qualifications do I need to become tenured?

Although qualifications for tenure may vary somewhat from institution to institution, the basic qualifications are remarkably similar. A primary qualification is a terminal degree in the area of teaching. In nursing, that is the doctoral degree. Some tenured nursing faculty do not possess the doctoral degree, but in most of these instances, tenure was granted many years ago when the master's degree was considered the terminal degree in nursing. Today, it is rare to find anyone hired for a tenure track position without a doctorate or significant progress toward that degree.

The remainder of the qualifications may be referred to in a variety of ways, but the essence of these categories speaks to the faculty member's teaching, scholarship, and service. The category of teaching is self-evident. Included in the teaching category is not only student evaluation of classroom teaching (although that is critically important), but also peer evaluations, participation in curriculum design, teaching innovations, curricular changes made in response to evaluations, and other activities that enhance student learning.

The category of scholarship may be narrowly or broadly defined. At a minimum, this category will include research activities, publications, and invited presentations. Research activities should clearly be related and demonstrate a planned program of research, building a particular body of knowledge within the discipline. Publications of most value in the tenure process are those in peer-reviewed journals that report findings of your research or synthesize the research of others in a particular area. While books, book chapters, and articles in nonreferred journals are useful in your tenure application, they do not carry the same weight.

Also included are invited presentations, especially those related to your research, at major conferences. Presentations usually need to be specified as to whether they were paper presentations or posters, and the nature of the conference specified (local, regional, national, international). Book reviews and leadership in a professional association may also be considered in this category at some institutions. (The chapter on research and scholarship provides a detailed discussion of related to this criterion.)

The category of service usually is divided into two sections. First is service to the college or university. This includes service within your department or division, but also (and especially!) service to the institution as a whole. While there are a variety of contributions one may make in this regard, service on committees at both levels is the more usual approach to satisfying this criterion. The second part of the service category is service to the community. Within this category is almost anything one does that is of benefit to the larger community: service on behalf of charitable organizations, public causes, political office, public committees, etc. At institutions where leadership in professional organizations is not included in the category for scholarship, it could be included with the area of community service. (See the chapter on faculty service activities for additional detail related to this criterion.)

8. How are my qualifications evaluated?

Evaluation of qualifications actually begins when you are hired. If you do not have the potential for meeting the qualifications, you will not be hired into a tenure track position. The rank at which you are hired also makes a difference in that the higher the rank, the greater the expectations of the institution when your tenure review is held.

Qualifications for tenure and promotion are published at each college and university in the faculty handbook or some other such document that describes the roles and responsibilities of faculty and administrations. A committee composed of faculty members from various disciplines within the university conducts a review of all materials submitted by faculty seeking tenure. The decision of this committee is then communicated to administration of the university.

The qualifications submitted by the applicant for tenure are usually in keeping with the categories described above; however, the relative weight given to each of the categories by members of the tenure review committee will vary from institution to institution. The weight given to each of the categories should be consistent with the college or university mission. Thus, if a college or university views itself primarily as a teaching institution, then the materials submitted in support of one's teaching will be heavily weighted. If, on the other hand, the university considers itself a research institution, then research, publications, grants, etc. may carry a higher weight than teaching. It is important as you prepare for tenure review to consider the relative importance of each category at your particular institution.

At many institutions, members of the tenure committee will hold an informational session to clarify the process at that particular college or university, and to describe any specifics of the tenure review that might be a preference at that institution. It is important for those considering applying for tenure to attend any such informational session that is offered. It is also appropriate, especially in the case where an informational session is not possible, to request a meeting with a member of the tenure review committee (usually the chair) to clarify any points of the process.

9. Other than the tenure committee, is there anyone else who can influence the tenure decision?

Of course, the person with the greatest influence in the tenure decision is the applicant, his or her readiness to seek tenure, the dossier constructed to support the tenure application, and the quality of the faculty member's own work. There are other people, however, who also are influential in the tenure process.

Once all the applicant's tenure materials are assembled, in most institutions they are made available for peer review. This review is, for the most part, limited to faculty of the same department, but there may be exceptions to this tradition for a variety of reasons. After reviewing the materials, each faculty member (usually those already tenured and holding a rank equal to or greater than that of the applicant) writes a letter to the tenure committee, sharing their opinion of the quality of the tenure candidate's performance according to the dossier and their knowledge of the applicant as a peer. These letters can be very influential in the tenure decision.

A letter is also written by the dean of the school or the department chairperson. This letter is similar to those of the faculty in that it speaks to the materials included in the tenure candidate's dossier, but also includes personal observations of the person's role and contributions as a faculty member, as an employee, and as an asset to the college or university. The letter from the dean or department chair also includes a recommendation to the tenure committee for granting or denying tenure. Although the decision is ultimately that of the tenure committee, the letters from the dean or department chair and faculty carry considerable weight.

Most colleges and universities also require that materials from the dossier be submitted for review to peers who are external to the institution. This element of the tenure process varies widely from institution to institution, although virtually all have an element of this process. In some instances the candidate is asked to submit the materials to external reviewers; in other situations, the candidate is asked to supply a list of names to the dean or department chair, who will then contact potential reviewers. In some situations the dean or department chair selects the external reviewers; in other instances, the tenure review committee makes the selection. It is important to know what the process is at your particular institution. External reviewers also submit letters/commentary that describe their evaluation of the materials they have reviewed. These reviews also carry considerable weight in the tenure decision-making process.

10. How do I prepare for tenure?

Preparation for tenure begins at the moment you are hired into a tenure track position, if not before. As you progress from day to day in your faculty role, tenure needs to be an ongoing consideration. Know the criteria upon which the tenure decision is based at your institution. Save everything that has to do with the categories described above. Most important, save student evaluations. Seek feedback and use it! Invite peers to come to your classes to give you an evaluation and constructive suggestions for improvement. Seek a mentor (see the chapter on mentoring to learn more about this). Keep records. Develop a program of research. Conduct research. Submit manuscripts to peer-reviewed journals. Apply for committees, both within the department and in the larger university. Participate in events on campus, recruitment events, and professional activities.

Begin, on the first day of your employment in a tenure track position, to create a "tenure file." Some faculty use a particular drawer in their file cabinet. Do not trust your memory to be able to recall what materials might be helpful and where those materials might be located. Save not only the successes, but also the attempts—for example, if you submit a grant application that is ultimately not funded or apply for a committee appointment that is not successful, keep these things for your tenure file. It shows your intent. If you have doubts as to whether something is germane to your tenure file, save it anyway. You can do the sorting when the time comes to create your dossier and to collect supporting materials.

11. What happens if I do achieve tenure?

Tenure brings with it a degree of job security and, perhaps more important, it safeguards academic freedom. Once tenure is granted, one's employment at the college or university can be terminated only for adequate cause, or under extraordinary circumstances, or because of the institution's severe financial need. Even in such circumstances, however, the faculty member has the right to initiate a grievance procedure.

Tenure does not mean, however, that faculty productivity and scholarly endeavors can cease. It becomes even more important for tenured faculty to mentor junior faculty and to serve as peer evaluators and role models for students and other faculty.

12. What happens if I don't achieve tenure?

If the tenure decision is negative, the faculty member to whom tenure has been denied may appeal the decision. While the right to appeal is virtually universal, there is variability as to the exact procedure from institution to institution. It is important to know the procedure in your university so that, should you receive a negative response, you can immediately launch an appeal. Your notification of intent to grieve the decision of the tenure committee may be on a very short time line. In addition, it is important to follow steps of the appeals process precisely.

If tenure is denied, the rationale for the decision must be available to the faculty member. This information may be helpful in the appeal process, but may also assist in preparation for another attempt at achieving tenure. In most institutions, a faculty member who is denied tenure is given the opportunity to reapply the following year. By using the information about the shortcomings or weak areas in the original tenure application, the faculty member can better attempt to clarify and strengthen the second application. The other choice in this situation is to seek a position at another college or university; one whose priorities for tenure may be a better fit for a particular faculty member.

13. What is meant by a tenure quota? How does it affect my chance for tenure?

While ideally, each faculty member's application for tenure would be judged solely on its own merits, there are institutions that explicitly or, more likely, implicitly, employ a quota system. Quota systems can be used in a variety of ways. For example, it may be the desire of the college or university that only a certain percentage of its faculty overall be tenured, or that only a certain percentage of each department's faculty be granted tenure, or that only a certain percentage of faculty be granted tenure each year.

It is difficult to state unequivocally just how an individual applicant might be affected by a quota system. However, it seems inherently flawed to have the tenure decision rest not with the quality of the applicant, but on factors that are beyond the applicant's control, such as the number of faculty in the department who have already been granted tenure, or the quantity and quality of applicants seeking tenure in the same year.

While seemingly unfair, colleges and universities that employ quota systems do so for two reasons: to remain intellectually vital and financially viable. Intellectual vitality depends, to some extent, on bringing in new faculty to the institution. Most institutions cannot afford to keep adding new faculty lines without proportionate increases in enrollment and revenue. Therefore, the institution counts on faculty positions becoming available as faculty move onto other positions or retire. Since faculty salaries comprise a major portion of a college or university's operating budget, it is in the institution's best interest to have faculty spread across the ranks. Having large numbers of faculty who are tenured means that these faculty are most likely in the top two ranks, associate professor and professor, where salaries are the highest and employment is, for the most part, guaranteed until retirement.

14. Why is there so much public sentiment against tenure?

In recent years the public discussion of the relative advantages and disadvantages of tenure has become more heated. There are several causes at the root of this anti-tenure sentiment. First, we as people may have become complacent about the magnitude of the danger to a free society posed by a loss of academic freedom in colleges and universities. Here in the United States, we cannot imagine our right to free speech being violated, and so we tend to take such freedoms for granted. A second reason may be envy. Most people do not have security in their jobs, and so, they argue, why should professors have such a benefit? The third reason is financial. In these days when boards of trustees are interested primarily in the "bottom line," tenured faculty are looked upon as a liability rather than an asset. The fourth reason lies with tenured faculty themselves, some of whom have become indifferent to the opportunities for creativity and scholarship and the challenges of the faculty role. This kind of faculty member, often referred to as "dead wood," does a great disservice to faculty colleagues by providing the negative stereotype so well used by those who would seek to end tenure.

15. What is post-tenure review?

Given the concerns described in the question above, some have suggested that a mechanism of post-tenure review is desirable, or even necessary, in order to maintain faculty productivity. In fact, most colleges and universities do have a system, usually within departments, where the dean or department chair evaluates the performance of faculty members on a regular basis. The content of the "performance review" varies from institution to institution; however, the essential elements remain: teaching, scholarship, and service. Recent discussions have taken the notion of periodic review of faculties' performance with the intent of constructive feedback and, thus, improvement, for the purpose of overriding a tenure decision if a faculty member is found lacking. This approach is viewed by many as an attempt to compromise the tenure system and a threat to academic freedom. Discussion on this topic is sure to continue.

16. What is the future of tenure?

Recent surveys of faculty are reported to show younger faculty as having a decreased interest in maintaining the present tenure system. There are several reasons why this may be so. Younger faculty have a vested interest in creation of more faculty openings. Because the present tenure system has been in place for the past 60 years, younger faculty may feel secure in the belief that academic freedom is inviolate and may not be able to envision the dangerous potential that would accompany its loss. Or they may sincerely believe in the benevolence of administration. It should be noted, however, that the overwhelming majority of faculty do indeed favor tenure.

Because of the financial implications of tenure, the tenure system is likely to be challenged regularly. As with anything that sustains continuous assaults, there will likely be some erosion. The United States Supreme Court has stated, "Our Nation is deeply committed to safeguarding academic freedom, which is of transcendent value to all of us and not merely to the teachers concerned. That freedom is, therefore, a special concern of the first amendment, which does not tolerate laws that cast a pall of orthodoxy over the classroom." I believe that practice of academic tenure will survive its many challenges, both internal and eternal, although the criteria for the granting of tenure may continue to become evermore demanding.

BIBLIOGRAPHY

1. Benedict ME, Wilder L: Unionization and tenure and rank outcomes in Ohio universities. J Labor Res 20:185, 1999.
2. Bess JL: Contract systems, bureaucracies, and faculty motivation: The probable effects of a no-tenure policy. J Higher Educ 69:1-22, 1998.
3. Park SM: Research, teaching, and service: why shouldn't women's work count? J Higher Educ 67:46-84, 1996.
4. Schoenfeld AC, Magnan R: Mentor in a Manual: Climbing the Academic Ladder to Tenure, 2nd ed. Madison, WI, Magna, 1994.
5. Williams J: The other politics of tenure. College Literature 26:226-237, 1999

IV. Issues and Teaching Strategies in Nursing Education

13. LEGAL AND ETHICAL ISSUES

Christine M. Henshaw, RN, MN, and Linda J. Scheetz, EdD, RN, CS, CEN

1. How do I know what is legal and ethical?

Many sources exist to help guide the professor's behavior. The International Council of Nurses Code of Ethics, written to guide the nurses' behavior with patients, is one place to start. Certainly, students should be treated with the same care and respect as patients. The National Education Association also has a Code of Ethics guiding faculty behavior. On a local level, your institution may have a code of ethics or ethical guidelines that guide faculty behavior.

In the legal arena, the nursing program and the college have policies that govern faculty actions. The registrar's office has policies regarding grading. The admissions office has policies regarding admissions. The nursing department may supplement these policies with departmental policies; however, those policies may not be in opposition to or in violation of the institution's policies. In the classroom, the syllabus guides the action. The college and the department may have student handbooks that state expected policies with regard to grading, absences, and so on. Problems arise when faculty or students fail to follow established published policies or procedures.

Public institutions generally have legal representation through the state's attorney general's office. Private institutions may have in-house counsel or may contract for legal services. Any question of a legal nature should move up the chain of command, all the way to the legal counsel as needed.

2. Who can I tell about my student's performance?

According to the Family Educational Rights Privacy Act (FERPA), commonly known as the Buckley Amendment, certain information about students is protected by federal law and may not be disclosed without the student's permission. FERPA does allow institutions to release information to the parents of a dependent child without prior consent of the student. Although certain "directory" information may be disclosed, dissemination of that information generally is funneled through one office on campus, for example, the registrar's office or the public information office. Even saying that a person is or is not a student in your class can be a problem. *Check your institution's policy, since your school may have a policy that is more restrictive than federal law.*

If a parent calls, seeking information about his or her child's performance in your course, *know your institution's policy before releasing any information!* As mentioned in the previous paragraph, institutions are permitted to establish policies that are more restrictive than federal law. If your college does NOT permit the release of information to the parent, inform the student of the parent's request, obtain the student's written permission to discuss his or her situation with the parents, then discuss only that information with the parents. If the student does not give permission, you will not be permitted to release information to the parents. If the student does give permission, it is probably a good idea to have the student present during the discussion with his parents.

3. Are students "working on my license"?

Professionals are responsible for their own actions. Students are also responsible for their actions. *You* are responsible for adequately preparing students for their role in patient care. Part of this responsibility is assigning students to perform only that care for which they have been properly prepared. Just as licensed practical nurses or certified nursing assistants are not working on your registered nurse license, students are not working on your license either.

Let's examine a hypothetical situation. Suppose that you are teaching students during their fourth quarter of clinical lab. Insertion of intravenous lines (IVs) is taught during this quarter, but not until later in the quarter. You inform students that they are not to start IVs until the principles have been discussed in theory class and practiced in the learning lab. The syllabus clearly identifies when IV insertion is taught, and also states that students are not to perform in clinical any skill they have not yet learned about in theory. In post-conference, you learn that a student attempted to start an IV on a patient before the procedure was taught in class and practiced in the lab. The student states, "The RN told me I should go ahead; she helped me." The IV start was not successful, and the patient had numbness and tingling in her hand after the attempt. She has notified her attorney. Are you at risk for a lawsuit?

While you may be named in a lawsuit, you have a good defense. Your syllabus clearly states that students should not perform procedures prior to learning about them, and you specifically called this to the student's attention. This student is acting outside his role, and is responsible for his own actions.

4. What do I do when students offer me gifts?

Although we all enjoy receiving gifts, it is probably best not to accept gifts of value from students. What is a gift of value? Your institution may have guidelines that spell out how much a gift may be worth. Absent that, it will be your discretion to determine whether or not a gift is acceptable. Gifts are problematic for many reasons. Depending on when they are given, they have the potential to influence grading decisions. If some students in your clinical section decide to give you a gift, others in the group may feel pressured into contributing even if they cannot afford it. Or some of the students in your clinical group may not wish to give a gift but feel peer pressure to contribute. A simple way to avoid this situation is to announce to students that you do not accept gifts.

5. Can my clinical students photocopy patients' records?

Students often ask to photocopy patients' records to ease their data collection process. Most clinical facilities prohibit this practice to maintain patient confidentiality. With new technologies, edges may become fuzzier as to what constitutes the patient record. For example, lab results may be printable from the computer. Even though those results are not physically in the patient's chart, they are considered part of the record and should not be copied or printed for students' use. Occasionally, facilities will allow students to copy records if the patient's name is obliterated. Extreme caution should be used and clear boundaries should be maintained so that students recognize this occasion as an exception. Always check the clinical agency's policy before permitting the student to copy or print any part of the patient's record.

6. What is my responsibility when a student makes an error in clinical?

Your first responsibility is to the patient. Address the patient's needs and ensure that the physician is notified according to facility policy. Complete the quality assurance or risk management report used by the facility. Confer with the student regarding the error, focusing on preventing further errors.

In addition, the school may have a report to complete, depending upon the nature of the incident. If the course is designed so that more than one faculty member is evaluating the student, notify the other faculty as needed. If the incident is serious or results in patient injury, notify the dean or director of the school of nursing.

7. How do I handle a student with a drug or alcohol problem?

The key is the student's *behavior*, regardless of the cause. Clear descriptions and expectations of student behavior, tied to clinical or classroom evaluation, allow you to make judgments based on the student's behavior. If the behavior is disruptive to the clinical or classroom situation, it is not acceptable. In the clinical setting, patient safety is always paramount. In the classroom, the needs of other students must be considered. Saying "This behavior violates policies" is more manageable than "I think you're on drugs; what are you taking?" Carefully document the unacceptable behavior and the consequences of such behavior. If the unacceptable behavior occurred in the clinical setting, also document any actual or potential harm to the patient as a result of the student's behavior. Be sure to document any conferencing done with the student, as well as your recommendations. A pattern of unacceptable behavior may result in course failure or disciplinary charges. Make sure the student has been informed in writing of the problem and the consequences of the behavior.

In areas with endemic drug and alcohol problems, faculty may investigate the possibility of random drug testing of students. This should be done in consultation with the school's legal counsel, and students should be notified of this practice prior to admission to the program.

8. What is educational malpractice and should I be concerned?

Educational malpractice, like medical malpractice, alleges injury from a breach of duty. With educational malpractice, the student alleges injury to the intellect or career from a failure to educate.[4] The student must prove the following elements to prevail in an educational malpractice suit:

- The educational institution owed a duty to the student to exercise reasonable care in the instruction and education of students.
- There was a breach of that duty.
- An injury resulted from the breach.
- There was damage to the student.[6]

Educational malpractice, however, is more difficult than medical malpractice to prove. Since there are many variables extraneous to the educational institution which influence learning, it is difficult for a student to prove that an injury resulted and that damage to the student occurred. Faculty's best defense is a good offense. Observe your school's policies; make course expectations and student responsibilities clear; prepare a written syllabus that includes the course description, objectives, content, grading procedures, and student responsibilities. Then, do your best job teaching the course and provide timely feedback to students about their progress in your course.

9. What if I am sued?

Anyone who follows the appropriate procedures may file a lawsuit. That does not mean that the suit has merit. As the American society becomes more litigious, faculty should not be surprised when students, also, file lawsuits. Although the institution may provide legal representation, you should consider retaining private counsel. The institution's attorney is hired to serve the interests of the institution; those interests may be in opposition to your own interests. If you believe that you need legal representation, professional educational associations may provide legal counsel to organization members.

Every effort should be made to resolve conflicts with students at the lowest possible level. If students are not satisfied at the faculty or department level, a grievance may be filed. If that does not resolve the issue, the student may decide to retain legal counsel. If you have any suspicion that the student has hired an attorney, the dean or director of the program should be notified. If the attorney contacts you directly, refer the attorney to the appropriate person(s) on your campus (for example, the university's attorney, the director of the program, the dean of students, or the registrar).

10. Why are student handbooks important?

Student handbooks are important because they include policy statements and other information pertinent to students. Student handbooks should be dated, reviewed periodically, and revised as needed. Documentation of the distribution of student handbooks should be maintained.

Many colleges and universities publish student handbooks for general populations of students, e.g., undergraduate students, graduate students. Additionally, nursing programs often publish student handbooks that are specific to their own students. Such handbooks should include policies and information that pertain specifically to nursing students. Consider adding a disclaimer to your handbook stating that the handbook is not a contract and the institution reserves the right to change policies with notice to students.

11. What student policies are important for nursing programs to have in place?

Policies can be categorized as those affecting all students in the institution and those affecting nursing students. *Institutional student policies* should address the following:

- Admission, progression, and retention
- Academic honesty/dishonesty
- Grade appeal
- Disability
- Acceptable use of academic computers
- Class attendance
- Student conduct (demonstrations, hazing, residence hall)
- Discrimination
- Sexual assault, rape, and harassment
- Drug and alcohol use/abuse
- Procedures for hearings

Also include a statement of how policy changes are made and promulgated.

Nursing-specific student policies should address the following:

- Expectations of student conduct in the clinical area
- Faculty's right to temporarily remove a student from a clinical setting without censure
- Clinical attendance
- Annual health examination and immunizations
- Grading, progression, and retention, if different for nursing students
- Advanced placement for RNs and LPNs

12. What should I do if a student violates a policy of the nursing program or the college?

Ideally, all policies of the nursing program and the college will be published and accessible to the academic community. Procedures for addressing policy violations should be published as well. Therefore, your first step should be to consult published handbooks or other policy manuals to seek direction in dealing with the problem. The next step should be notification of the appropriate administrator (dean of students or dean of nursing). Do not take any action against the student until you are clear about the policy and the procedure to follow when the policy has been violated. An exception to this rule would be student behavior in the clinical setting which jeopardizes patient safety, i.e., gross negligence or practicing under the influence of alcohol or mind-altering drugs. In cases where patient safety is jeopardized, the student should be removed from the clinical area immediately. Then, refer to policy manuals, handbooks, or the dean to find out what the next step is.

The student should be informed in writing of the specific violation and the implications of such. The student should have the opportunity to respond to the charge(s) and to submit any mitigating circumstances. Unless the policy indicates otherwise, a hearing may be scheduled, during which the charge(s) against the student will be presented. At this time, the student will have the opportunity to respond to the charge(s). Such hearings are administrative, rather than judicial, in nature. Students are usually permitted to have counsel present (legal or academic). However, whether or not counsel will be permitted to participate in the hearing in any capacity other than that of an adviser to the student should be determined beforehand and be consistent with established college policy.

13. What is due process and how does it impact my dealings with students?

Due process is a constitutional right of every individual in this country; however, it can mean different things in different situations. Constitutional due process intends to protect individuals from unfair government interference. Public institutions (e.g., state colleges and universities) are considered agents of the government. However, independent colleges and universities are not agents of the government and thus have more freedom in determining due process. Independent institutions, therefore, establish their own definition of due process. However, once the institution defines due process and related procedures, these must be adhered to. Since many legal issues in higher education involve fairness and adherence to contractual policies, disputes that arise between students and the institution relate to the contract established between the student and the institution. To resolve these disputes in the legal arena, courts examine the contract between the student and the institution, considering the issue of due process as it relates to the type of institution.

There are two types of due process: procedural and substantive. Procedural due process means that *procedures* (e.g., the rules) used in academic decision making are fair and impartial. An example of procedural due process is allowing the student to appear before a panel or committee to hear the charges against him or her and to respond to the charges. Substantive due process is concerned with the outcome of the academic decision, and whether it is fair and reasonable. To make a decision against the student which is grounded in prejudice, or is otherwise arbitrary or capricious, constitutes denial of substantive due process.

When making academic decisions, faculty and administrators should be cognizant of both procedural and substantive due process as defined by the institution. Some examples of procedural due process might include the following:

- The charges against the student are presented in writing in understandable language.
- The charges are presented within a reasonable time of the alleged policy violation.
- The student is provided with an opportunity to respond to the charges and to be heard by an impartial committee or panel convened for this purpose.
- The student is permitted the right to counsel.

Examples of substantive due process are:

- Only information permitted at the hearing is considered in deciding the outcome of the charges.
- Personal bias is set aside by those involved in determining the outcome.
- Decisions about the outcome are rational and consistent with information presented at the hearing.

Clearly, careful attention to the development and writing of policies and procedures is vital to ensure they are clear, legal, and useful to the student and the institution. Due process procedures should be published and accessible to the academic community. Because published documents define the nature of the contract between the student and the institution, published policies and procedures should be followed to the letter.

14. What are my legal and ethical responsibilities regarding letters of recommendation for students?

Letters of recommendation become a legal and ethical issue for faculty when faculty have information that may not present the student in a positive light to potential employers or graduate school admission committees. From a legal perspective, faculty who state in writing information that the student perceives to cast him or her in a negative light run the risk of a lawsuit by the student for defamation of character. From an ethical perspective, faculty who withhold negative information that relates to the position applied for quite possibly violate ethical principles related to beneficence (e.g., do no harm, as in patient welfare).

So, how do you reconcile legal and ethical responsibilities and keep everyone happy? The best approach is one of truthfulness from the start. If you feel that your letter of recommendation will not place the student in a positive light or may jeopardize the student's ability to secure a job or graduate school admission, tell the student at the time of the request. That puts the ball back into the student's court. He or she can then withdraw the request for a letter of reference. Courts have ruled that letters of recommendation, written for students by faculty, for the specific purpose for which they were intended, do not meet the legal standard for defamation of character. If your letter of recommendation meets the following conditions, it is unlikely that the student will prevail in a defamation lawsuit:

- Written at the *written* request of the student
- Directed only to the individual specified by the student
- Written for the purpose specified by the student (e.g., recommendation for employment or graduate school)
- Presents your fair and honest appraisal of the student's ability, performance, and potential
- Includes an accurate representation of the facts

To avoid allegations of breach of privacy, require that the student submit to you a detailed written request for a letter of reference. Keep the student's request on file.

15. How should I handle a student who I believe has cheated in a class assignment or on an exam?

Clarify in your own mind what you believe the student did that constituted cheating. Did the student

- Use a crib sheet during an exam?
- Engage in a signal answer system with other students during an exam?
- Collaborate with another student to write a paper?
- Copy answers to an exam from another student's test?

Once you have a clear sense of the student's behavior and the outcome of that behavior, it is time to meet *privately* with the student. Rather than outrightly accusing the student of cheating, you might try this approach, "Bill, I noticed that the answers on your test and Lisa's test were exactly the same, including the incorrect answers. Help me to understand how that happened. My records indicate that Lisa was sitting in front of you." Then, wait for a response. Silence is your friend! If the student did indeed cheat, he or she may be so uncomfortable by your statement and the following period of silence that a confession is forthcoming. If the student admits cheating, you should proceed by following the institution's academic dishonesty policy. Most policies allow for a range of punishment, depending upon the seriousness of the violation. Faculty will often opt to assign a failing grade for the test or paper or for the entire course. If the student denies cheating and you are convinced that it occurred, implement the institutional policy, which often means that allegations must be presented in writing, followed by a hearing, if the issue remains unresolved between the you and student.

16. How should I handle a student who I believe has falsified records in the clinical setting?

Many colleges and universities consider falsification of records a form of academic dishonesty. Many nursing programs also consider such behavior to be fraudulent practice and, as such, may be addressed by your nursing program's policy for student conduct in the clinical setting. Your first step is to clarify the behavior in light of your institution's academic dishonesty and clinical conduct policies.

Begin as you would if you suspected the student of cheating in the classroom. Ask and answer these questions: "What did the student do to make me suspect falsification? What documentation do I have to support this allegation?" If you have a clear picture of what the student did and the documentation to support your allegations, it is time to meet *privately* with the student. Share your information with the student. For example, if the student charted a medication as given, which, in fact, was not given, present this information to the student. Try this approach: "Susan, you signed the medication administration record, indicating that you administered furosemide to Mrs. Jones at 10:00 a.m. When I spoke with Mrs. Jones, she told me that you had not given her any medication this morning. When I checked the medication drawer, Mrs. Jones' 10:00 a.m. dose of furosemide was in the drawer. Help me to understand why you charted that you had administered this drug." This approach alerts the student that you have conflicting information and are requesting clarification. If the student *erroneously* charted that the medication had been given, you will most likely proceed differently than you would if the student had intentionally falsified the record. If it turns out that the student *intentionally falsified* the record, inform the dean of nursing and file appropriate charges according to your institution's policy. You will also need to inform the nurse manager of the unit on which the error or falsification occurred.

If you suspect falsification of records but do not have irrefutable documentation, you should confront the student with your suspicions anyway. However, you may not want to file formal charges at this time. The student should be advised that such behavior will not be tolerated and that charges are pending. Before bringing formal charges against the student, make certain that you have adequate documentation from reliable sources to support the charges. Implement whatever policies apply and follow the policies to the letter.

17. What are my legal responsibilities to students regarding the Americans with Disabilities Act (ADA)?

Your legal responsibilities are to provide reasonable accommodations to the student, provided the student has documented that his or her disability warrants such accommodation under the ADA. If a student requests accommodations, you should contact your institution's disabilities officer to determine whether the institution has satisfactory documentation for the disability and, if so, what accommodations are reasonable. The issue of providing reasonable accommodations for students in the clinical setting is not as well-defined as it is for the on-campus setting. When considering what accommodations might be reasonable, especially for the clinical area, keep in mind that the law does not mandate lower standards or compromises in safety, just reasonable accommodations. The goal of the ADA is to provide disabled students the same opportunity as nondisabled students to complete an academic program. (Refer to the chapter "Students with Special Needs" for more information on this topic.)

18. What are the legal implications of evaluating students, particularly in the clinical setting?

Most students are intimidated by faculty evaluations of their performance, and justifiably so. After all, decisions that faculty make about students' performance have far-reaching effects that impact students' careers. When students are judged to have failed, entry into the chosen career may be delayed or never realized. Thus, faculty have an ethical and legal responsibility to make the most objective, accurate, and logical decisions about students' performance that are possible. When faculty deviate from such a standard, they subject themselves to potential litigation.

The legal issues with evaluation usually relate to objectivity and fairness, especially where clinical evaluation is concerned. Therefore, it is imperative that all evaluation processes are as objective and free of bias and measurement error as possible. Students should be informed at the beginning of the semester how they will be evaluated and how each evaluation measure (exams, papers, clinical evaluation) will be weighted to calculate the final course grade. Students also should be informed at the beginning of the clinical experience of the performance standards against which they will be evaluated.

19. Are there any other legal issues that I should be concerned with as a faculty member?

There are any number of legal issues that can arise between students and faculty. Courts have been reluctant to interfere with academic decision making, while choosing instead to focus on the contract between the student and the institution, due process, and issues of good faith and fairness. Because faculty have wide latitude in academic decision making, it is always advisable to act in good faith, with sound educational rationale, and to apply policies and procedures fairly and consistently. While students may not like the outcome, if you have acted with good intentions and made decisions that are rational and objective, rather than arbitrary and capricious, you will probably have little to worry about.

Areas of Legal Concern to Faculty

CONCERN	ISSUE	COMMENTS
Grading policies	Student claims lack of knowledge about how his grade is determined; inconsistent grading among students.	Policy should be published and adhered to; apply equitably
Cancellation of classes or major changes in course syllabus after course begins	Student claims that he did not get what was paid for.	Make every attempt to adhere to the course schedule and description; changes should be justified by acceptable educational rationale.
Incorrect academic advisement	A type of estoppel, where the student follows faculty advice that is erroneous; as a consequence, does not fulfill graduation requirements as anticipated.	Become thoroughly familiar with all program and institutional requirements for graduation. If you make an error, inform the student and dean immediately. Be an advocate for the student in attempting to correct the error and resolve the situation.

Continued on following page.

Areas of Legal Concern to Faculty (Continued)

CONCERN	ISSUE	COMMENTS
Changing academic requirements	Student claims that he or she was delayed or prevented from graduating because of changing requirements; claims that changing requirements present undue hardship	Include a disclaimer in catalogs and handbooks, giving the institution the right to change requirements. Always promulgate in writing any change in requirements. Implement a change in academic requirements to minimize disruption in academic progress for students; only change requirements when academically justified.
Defamation (comments about students)	Faculty make negative comments about a student; student claims defamation (oral, slander; written, libel)	Negative comments/evaluation about/of students should be supported by legitimate academic reasons and made only to those with a legitimate need to know.[6]

BIBLIOGRAPHY

1. International Council of Nurses: Code for Nurses (Online) 1999, http://icn.ch/publications.htm#classics
2. Kaplin WA, Lee BA: The Law of Higher Education: A Comprehensive Guide to Legal Implications of Administrative Decision Making, 3rd ed. San Francisco, Jossey-Bass, 1995.
3. National Education Association: Code of Ethics of the Education Profession (Online) 1999. http://www.nea.org/aboutnea/code.html
4. Rupert PA, Holmes DL: Dual relationships in higher education. J Higher Educ 68:660-678, 1997.
5. Stoner EN, Detar CA: Disciplinary and academic decisions pertaining to students in higher education. J College Univ Law 26: 273-90, 1999.
6. Weeks KM: Faculty Decision Making and the Law. Nashville, College Legal Information, Inc., 1994.
7. Weeks KM: Managing Departments: Chairpersons and the Law. Nashville, College Legal Information, Inc., 1996.
8. Helms LB, Weiler K: Disability discrimination in nursing education: an evaluation of legislation and litigation. J Prof Nurs 9:358-366, 1993.

14. CONCERNS OF AND ABOUT STUDENTS

Elizabeth N. Stokes, PhD, RN, Geraldine Valencia-Go, PhD, RN, CS,
and Kelly Fisher, MS, RN

1. Students sometimes begin to tell me about problems of a personal nature. The problems, although they affect academic/clinical performance, are outside the realm of academic counseling. The problems are real, but I am uncomfortable dealing with these revelations. What should I do?

Good question, and one that arises frequently when students perceive faculty as approachable and sensitive to their needs and concerns. However, the help that such students require is beyond the teacher-student relationship, so it is important to stop students' revelations. Be careful when communicating this to students, since you don't want to appear insensitive. Validate that the students' problems are real. Demonstrate sympathy for the situation. Caution students that they may not want to reveal this information to a faculty member. Recommend that students find someone not involved with their studies to help them deal with the problem. Try to get the student to some kind of counseling. Give the student specific information about resources. You may need to provide information about what counseling will do, what counseling is like, and what the student should expect. Often students think needing/going to counseling is a sign of weakness or "being crazy." Emphasize the benefits of a neutral person's perspective.

2. What if the student is in a crisis situation? What should I do?

Depending upon the degree of crisis, you may call the counseling center from your office to help the student set up the initial appointment. If the situation is an emergency or you think there is potential for immediate self-harm, you may accompany the student to the counselor's office. If the counselor is not available, arrange for transportation to the emergency department. The student should not be left alone. If you cannot accompany the student, ask someone from the security department or student services staff to do so.

3. What information do I need in order to refer students to counseling services?

It is extremely important that teachers be familiar with resources in their schools and community. You should also be aware of what fees may be associated with counseling. Many schools provide short-term counseling without charge. The Student Services Office or the Dean of Students' Office should have this information. Such information is usually published in student handbooks, also.

4. I have been trained as a therapist; what should I do about counseling students?

If you are a trained therapist, counseling current and/or prospective students is ill-advised as long as you are a teaching faculty member. The phases of the counseling relationship could potentially interfere with the student-faculty relationship. Potential problems include allegations of favoritism, feelings of manipulation, and inclinations toward protectionism.

5. The idea of counseling baffles me, but I know this is important. What steps should I take to be more comfortable in this area?

Discuss your feelings with an experienced faculty (or an assigned faculty mentor, if you have one). While you will not be involved in student counseling, you should feel comfortable discussing available services with students. Become informed about counseling services available for students. If there are several faculty who share your discomfort, ask the faculty member with a psychiatric/mental health background to hold an information session for you. If you are alone in your discomfort with this situation, perhaps a one-on-one meeting with a psychiatric/mental health faculty colleague or campus counselor will alleviate your concerns.

6. I want to be approachable as a teacher, but am afraid of being too friendly. What advice would you give about faculty-student relationships?

The student-faculty relationship is a work relationship. Faculty are perceived as authority figures; therefore, students may be intimidated by faculty. A feeling of overwhelming intimidation by faculty usually interferes with learning, so try to avoid intimidating students. Faculty are responsible for establishing the structure for teaching-learning, the standards for accomplishing objectives, and the rules of the course. You can be friendly with students without establishing an intense social relationship. In the beginning of your course or clinical, you may invite students to share some personal information, such as hometown and why they chose nursing. You may ask students to tell a favorite subject, a hobby, or something others would be unlikely to know. If you do this kind of introduction or "icebreaker," you should also share about yourself. This sharing makes you seem more "human." Sharing break or meal times or talking with students during class breaks are other ways that make you approachable. Some faculty bring food for discussion groups, the last class/group meeting, or an early morning class. These are instances of involving all of a clinical group or class. You have to decide what your feelings are about such situations. Some faculty prefer more distance from students. Others are comfortable with a closer but somewhat casual approach to students.

Problems arise when faculty establish close social relationships with students, especially at the undergraduate level. Such situations are very problematic when such friendships involve only one or two students from a group or class. Some schools have policies governing student-faculty relationships.

7. Some students seem very dependent upon faculty or expect faculty to tell them how to proceed. I think students should be able to start a paper or an assignment or plan for patient care without me telling them every step. What do I do about the dependent student?

After the careful explanations of the guidelines you have established, ask the student for additional questions. If the level of the student and the tone of the questions are inappropriate in terms of independence, you might start by asking questions of the student. Try using some of the examples listed below.
- What do you think this guideline means?
- What would you tell someone about this assignment?
- What ideas do you have about the assignment?
- What reading have you done?
- Tell me about a problem you encountered or observed in the clinical area.
- What clinical experience have you had with a client with similar problems? What did you do? What was the outcome?

Suggest that the student write a list of ideas or an outline for you to discuss and review. For students who appear to want you to do a plan of care, suggest that they complete specified work (for instance, two problems, a priority problem with interventions) and then discuss it with you. Also, setting time limits may be appropriate for some students.

8. I am worried that students will make a mistake in clinical. I want to be sure that students know what they are doing. How do I find a "happy medium" between being too cautious and letting the students do things on their own?

Develop a system of checks and balances. It helps to develop your own system of keeping up with the assigned client and student information. Require preparation for the clinical setting with specific expectations. Let students know when you expect to be with them for certain procedures or skills. For new skills or procedures infrequently performed, review the procedure with the student before seeing the client. Checking closely with students at the beginning of a clinical experience will give you an idea about the capabilities of students. If your program uses a checklist of clinical experiences, review the list at the beginning of the experience and periodically during the experience.

You want to may develop a checklist or survey of your own. Make a list of clinical experiences including skills available in your area. Structure your survey with choices such as have performed many times, performed once or twice, and never performed, or, much experience, little experience, no experience. You may also ask students what their needed experiences are, what they would like to learn. Again, check with students during the experience to determine the status of their performance or experiences. Students become very frustrated if asked about needed experiences but the instructor appears to make little effort to help students gain these experiences.

9. What about correcting students in front of clients (and their families)?

Correcting students in front of clients may jeopardize the rapport the student has established with the client. Certainly the correction diminishes both client and student confidence. Find a way to use the student's communication or performance to provide correct information or to change the performance.

Strategies that you can use to change or correct what may be erroneous or partially incorrect information are identified below.

State to the student:
- "Let me help you with . . . Sometimes a third hand is useful."
- "I will be your assistant. If we move this way, we will be more efficient."
- "I think we can accomplish this by doing this. Let's see if this is effective."

State to the patient:
- "The student is on the right track. Emphasis should be placed on . . ."
- "The student is trying to comfort (reassure) you. This is obviously a trying time for you. You said you were concerned about . . ."

Finally, model appropriate communication to validate legitimate feelings of the client. Outside the client's hearing, discuss with the student problems that arise with false reassurance. When you're alone with the student, repeat your communication as an example of therapeutic communication.

10. How can I avoid making comments or asking questions that appear to "make fun of," belittle, or demean students about their knowledge or performance? Students often say they are afraid to ask questions because the faculty member labels their questions as dumb.

Nursing students are often lacking in self-confidence. Sarcasm, labeling, derision, and ridicule have no place in student-faculty communication. Demonstrate respect for the student in both verbal and nonverbal communication. If the student asks a question that seems "dumb," the question is a manifestation of a lack of understanding. Give a legitimate answer to the question. In face-to-face communication, you can check verbally or nonverbally the student's grasp of information. If you think the student lacks specific information, a private discussion with the student will help determine the extent of the problem. Remember, your goal as faculty is to facilitate learning.

A wise and learned teacher often said, "If the student or whoever has a question, learning did not take place in the past on this topic. Learning, however, can take place now." This teacher's approach was not to blame anyone for lack of knowledge and to facilitate acquiring the knowledge now. If lack of information surfaces as a group problem, you may want to investigate the area as a curriculum problem. Such an approach also frees faculty to solve the problem rather than defend what they may or may not have taught.

11. What about questions or explanations involving one or two students that take an extended amount of time, especially in the classroom?

If the majority of the class is ready to move on, it is appropriate to ask the involved students to meet after class for addition information or explanation. It is a good idea to check with the entire class about their understanding of the topic at the beginning of the next class period.

12. What about students who either monopolize discussions or ask questions that are off the topic?

Ask the student to meet privately with you. Be careful not to silence the student. Acknowledge that the student is thinking or has read extensively or had more experience, or whatever. You have some options to discourage such behavior. If this happens frequently, try limiting the number of questions each student may ask per discussion or class period. Tell the student who monopolizes that if others have not had a chance to discuss or ask questions, you will ask that she or he let others speak before making another comment or asking a second question.

For off-the-topic questions, meet with the student privately. Do not belittle or demean the student, but acknowledge that student is thinking or you are pleased that the student has explored this area. Communicate to the student that the class is not always at the same level. Tell students that you may not answer all questions in class. Offer to remain after class for 5 minutes or so to answer questions. Then, be sure to follow through with your plan.

13. Some students in my school have lifestyles or cultures very different from mine. I observe some behaviors that are not a part of my personal belief system or are different from my own upbringing. What are some suggestions for working with these students?

You have started working positively with students who differ from you in some way by acknowledging the differences. Is the behavior, lifestyle, or belief system harmful in some way to the care of clients? Policies of clinical agencies may govern certain practices, such as body piercing, for example. Is the student trying to impose his or her belief on you or clients? Your response to the student should be on the basis of his or her achievement rather than a lifestyle.

If the student belongs to a different culture, obtain information from both the student and the literature about the beliefs, attitudes, customs, and practices of the culture. Discuss expectations related to clinical experiences with the student prior to the first day of clinical. Try to make adaptations within the course or clinical that will allow the student to practice his or her customs.

The following anecdote describes the experience of a student whose practices differed from those of the majority:

A nursing student belonged to a group that did not cut their hair, wore natural fiber clothing, did not eat meat, and bathed but did not use deodorants. The student talked with instructors about these practices. He always tied his hair back very neatly, but sometimes his body odor would become offensive. He became more meticulous about bathing before coming to the clinical area. The student would also check with students in the group who would be honest with him about his body odor. He gained permission to use facilities in a clinical agency for extra showers.

For further information on teaching students from different cultures, turn to the discussion in the chapter on teaching to a diverse student group.

14. Students learn in different ways. How can I teach when there is such diversity of student learning styles?

Learning modes include auditory, visual, and tactile. Students may be more comfortable with one mode of learning than another. Some students want to experiment with teaching equipment, such as that used in the lab. These are students who want to "go first." Others prefer to observe before trying out a new skill. In the classroom, using several types of stimuli at once helps all students with learning. The student hears a voice (or a sound track) and sees illustrations or pictures. The instructor may have pieces of equipment for students to handle. Choosing books that have readable text as well as useful pictures and diagrams also addresses different learning style preferences.

Concept mapping is another way of helping students learn complex material. Students visualize relationships between concepts by drawing diagrams. For example, the student might create a concept map on blood coagulation. Later, the student could add anticoagulant drugs to the area on the concept map where the action of these drugs occurs. Concept maps, constructed by students, aid knowledge recall and organization. (More about this in the chapter on Critical Thinking!)

15. What about students for whom English is a second language?

Students should have met a specified requirement for use of both oral and written English. Even so, many such students continue to have a language difficulty. Learning colloquialisms as well as the language of health care means that these students are trying to learn to use four languages (native tongue, correct English, colloquial terms, and health care language). You would be confused, too! The writer (Stokes) was told by a person with expertise with international students that generally the grades earned by such students were one letter grade below their true capability.

16. What are some practical strategies for helping nonnative English speakers with language?

Suggest that students form a buddy system or work with a study group. The buddy or study group should have students for whom English is the native language. Carrying translation dictionaries is also helpful.

Advise students to keep a separate page and write down words/phrases from class or books that are not understood. The instructor should work with the student initially on the word list. Students may also work with their buddy or study group on language that is not clear.

17. What about testing for nonnative English speakers?

Students for whom English is a second language often misunderstand or read questions incorrectly. Some instructors permit the more novice students to use a translation dictionary during a test. A translation dictionary gives the word in the native tongue and in English.

No definition is provided. This writer (Stokes) has had success with permitting students to take the test in a room with the instructor. (Special scheduling was used to accomplish this.) The student was permitted to ask questions about test items. The student could ask about words or validate that she or he had the meaning of question or distractor correct. If the explanation would give away the answer, the student was told that the instructor was unable to answer. As the student gains more experience with the English language, such arrangements may not be necessary.

Note that all variations of English are not the same. This writer (Stokes) has had experience with students from Great Britain or its former colonies who spoke absolutely wonderful, very elegant, and grammatically correct English, but misinterpreted the meaning of "Americanisms," colloquial English, or medical "Americanese" jargon.

18. What is team teaching? What contributes to the success of team teaching?

Team teaching involves one or more faculty teaching in the same course. Team teaching is often done when more than one specialty area is represented in an undergraduate course, when content is very heavy, or when the number of credit hours is high. Course content is divided among faculty on the teaching team. Usually each faculty member is responsible for specific classes, learning activities, and testing for their content areas.

Team teaching in clinical experiences is a common practice. Several faculty may be involved in clinical experiences for one course. Students may have common clinical conferences and/or individual clinical conferences with their faculty. The objectives of the clinical course are the same for all students. Faculty remain in a specific clinical area, and students may rotate between several clinical areas within one course. The advantage of rotating students among faculty for a clinical experience is that more than one faculty member contributes to the evaluation of the student. This is especially helpful if a student's performance is marginal, since input from more than one faculty member probably provides greater objectivity.

19. What steps can be taken to ensure that team teaching is successful? Who is in charge of the course?

Coordination and planning are essential to the success of team teaching. A course coordinator should be assigned to each course. This assignment may rotate among faculty. The coordinator is responsible for bringing the group together and directing the course. Coordinators may be responsible for putting the course syllabus together. Meetings with the faculty team are important. Planning meetings should be held prior to the beginning of the term, often in the previous term, or before school ends for the summer. Regular meetings throughout the term provide the opportunity for questions, progress reports, and discussion of problems.

20. What about planning for team teaching?

Planning meetings are especially important. Course objectives, specific requirements, and expectations are reviewed. The background of the students in relation to the content should be discussed. Testing in the classroom must be coordinated. A test blueprint should be devised by the course coordinator or by group consensus. The course coordinator should set deadlines so tests can be assembled, word-processed, proofed, copied, and ready for distribution. Team faculty, in some instances, review and revise test questions as a group.

Clinical coordinators and faculty may discuss the level of the students and expectations. If some faculty are new to the course, previous courses and experiences of students should be delineated. Evaluation tools should be explained. If completed sample evaluation tools from previous courses are available, a review of these tools may be helpful. More experienced faculty may give examples of student experiences or specific information about expectations to assist newer faculty with their integration into the course.

21. What are some ways to manage courses that involve team teaching?

Periodic meetings may be held to discuss the course. Relative to content, discussions may revolve around testing, student preparation, student response and progress relative to learning activities, and classroom policies. As indicated, some teaching teams review and revise test questions. Relative to clinical learning experiences, the team may discuss implementation of course guidelines, student progress problems, strategies that are successful, the quantity and quality of learning experiences, and the quality of student work.

22. Students sometimes complain about inconsistency among faculty. The crux of the matter is that faculty have different teaching styles. What advice or explanation may be given to students?

Differences are a fact of life. Both teaching and learning styles may differ. While faculty may work at being consistent about requirements and expectations, some differences remain. Faculty should seriously consider student feedback about inconsistencies and try to rectify differences in requirements or expectations. Consistency about absences, tardiness, and lack of preparation should be maintained throughout the course. Work requirements for students at the same level should be fair. Guided discussion with faculty and students may alleviate some student complaints. Discussion at the beginning of the term/course/clinical to remind students about variations in people, content, learning, and teaching may be helpful. Explanations that include levels of content difficulty, levels of expectations, and required knowledge (one should have more knowledge about common health problems than rare diseases) may be useful. Analogies (e.g., choices of friends, likes and dislikes, study habits, favorite subjects, and preferred colors) may be useful in stimulating the thinking of students.

Try drawing a parallel to clinical experiences. Client behaviors are sometimes harmful. All clients are not cheerful, thankful, or friendly. Future work settings will be populated with co-workers with various work styles, and personalities. Future bosses will have different management styles. In a nutshell, while faculty should strive to be consistent in their expectations of students and standards for student performance, they should also assist students to accept and appreciate diversity among faculty, just as students should accept and appreciate diversity among peers and patients.

23. What should I do about the student who is performing poorly in the clinical area?

Clinical objectives and expectations should be explicitly clear. The student who is less than satisfactory (as well as students who are doing satisfactorily) should have immediate feedback. The conference between the student who is performing poorly and the instructor should be private. Restate objectives and expectations. Provide specific information about the poor performance. Ask the student to self-evaluate clinical performance. Determine, if possible, the cause of the poor performance. Does the student need more practice with skills? Is the student not applying content appropriately in the clinical area? Is this reflective of a lack of knowledge? Is the clinical difficulty a problem of knowledge transfer? Formulate a plan or contract that will enable the student to achieve a satisfactory performance. Both the student and the instructor should have a copy of the plan. Document the poor performance and your conference with the student. (More on this topic in the chapters "Clinical Teaching" and "Student Evaluation".)

24. What about the student who continues to fail in the classroom or in the clinical area?

Timely feedback to the student is essential. Document conferences with the student. Many schools have a form for this purpose. Recommendations, advice, and plans for remedying the situation may be included. Any information given to the student should be included. For example, the instructor reiterates that all test grades are in the failure range and that continuation in the course will result in a grade of F.

A copy of the form is given to the student, and the instructor retains a copy. Students may be required to sign the form to acknowledge that they have received the information. The instructor should document all interactions with the student. Depending on the situation, the course/level coordinator or the department chair should be informed about the situation.

25. What about the student who earns a grade of F? What if the student appeals the grade?

Information about the meaning of a failure should be given orally to the student. The student should also be directed to written policies about failures. In many programs, two failures result in dismissal from the program. If the student is dissatisfied about the grade, the student has a right to appeal. The student should receive information about the proper procedure to follow for appealing a grade.

The instructor should gather information regarding the student's performance. Although grade appeals are not pleasant experiences, the instructor who has thoroughly documented the performance of the student, efforts to help the student, and conferences regarding the problems will be well-prepared for the grade appeal proceeding. (Refer to the chapter "Legal and Ethical Issues" for additional information about this topic.)

26. What about substance abuse by nursing students?

Nurses and nursing students are vulnerable to substance abuse. Remember, substance abuse includes alcohol as well as drugs. Students experience stress and may seek relief in unhealthy ways. Using pills to stay up to study, then pills to go to sleep, and pills to stay calm can quickly become a habit. Education about substance abuse is usually included in most nursing curricula. However, neither students nor faculty view the vulnerability and risk of substance abuse from a personal perspective. The writer (Stokes) suggests that an excellent student-sponsored program would be a talk from an impaired but recovering health care worker.

27. How should the topic of substance abuse be managed?

The nursing program should establish a substance abuse policy. If the program does not have such a policy, gather information from colleagues in other schools. Talk to local clinical agencies. Many clinical agencies have viable policies. Personnel in clinical agencies who are responsible for policy implementation are often good resources for educating faculty and/or students about substance abuse. Faculty with psychiatric/mental health backgrounds possess a wealth of information in this area.

28. What about substance abuse policies?

Most colleges/universities have a substance/drug abuse policy. Such policies may not be useful in the health care area. Faculty are particularly concerned about the possibility of substance abuse affecting clinical performance and the potential harm such abuse presents to clients. After establishing substance abuse policies, policies should be widely distributed and discussed. Orientation to substance abuse policies should include both faculty and students. Some orientation programs include a short quiz to determine if faculty/students have sufficient knowledge about substance abuse policies.

29. My program has a substance abuse policy, but it is a bit involved. How can I remember what behaviors to observe and what to do if I suspect substance abuse?

Review the substance abuse policy and procedures at least once a term. If team teaching is the norm, the course coordinator or a designee should review the policies and procedures during planning meetings. Several faculty who work with the writer (Stokes) include a copy of the substance abuse policy and procedures with information (on a clipboard or in a folder) carried to the clinical area. Faculty should be knowledgeable about behaviors that might be manifestations of substance abuse. If an incident involving substance abuse does occur, faculty should follow prescribed procedures. Required documentation should be completed promptly. Actions taken should be reported to the course coordinator, department chair, and/or dean/director of the nursing program.

30. Describe an effective classroom strategy that gives students an incentive to prepare prior to class and maintains their attention and involvement.

Most nursing students have multiple commitments and have difficulty preparing prior to class. However, when students are given incentives that they know will improve their performance and hence, grades, they are usually receptive to realigning their priorities. A strategy that has worked effectively starts with a teaching-learning contract that outlines the responsibilities of the faculty and students. This contract is reviewed, signed, and retained by both.

One aspect of the contract entails the submission of a critical thinking log. Students would need to do the reading assignments prior to class. There are three areas to be addressed:

• Express in 3-4 sentences the main concept(s) discussed in the chapter.
• Express in 3-4 sentences the most important information you learned.
• My concerns or questions about the material are. . .

Students submit this one-page log at the beginning of class. Faculty should take few minutes during class or break time to review the three areas, especially the third one. These areas establish the basis for class discussions. Ten minutes before the end of each class, students complete the second part of the log that asks the following:

• The additional learning I obtained from the class includes. . .
• Further questions I will ask about the material are. . .
• After today, I will use the information in the following ways. . .

The incentive part of the strategy is directly related to the log. At the beginning of the course, each student takes a card with a number and writes her or his name on it. The cards are then kept in a sealed envelope. A corresponding set of index cards with only numbers is created by the faculty. These cards get shuffled during class discussion. Because the faculty member does not know which student has a given number, every student has the potential for being called upon during the class discussion. Students get additional points added to their final course grade for every correct response they give. Absences are rare, and everyone vies to answer questions. Every class is an exciting, fun-filled exchange between students and faculty. An additional advantage of the log is that it provides an opportunity to assess students' writing skills and level of critical thinking.

Students who have participated in this strategy reported better understanding of content and improved time management. Students also found that they made time to do their readings in order to write the log. As a result, they felt more adequately prepared for examinations. The faculty and course evaluations were extremely positive and students' grades were the best ever the first year that this strategy was implemented.

31. How can I curb complaints related to the preparation work for clinical?

Approach clinical preparation as a learning activity to meet two specific goals:

• A requirement for delivering competent patient care
• Preparation for the clinical examination

Students could complete the same critical thinking logs as described in the previous question. In addition, students are asked to create notes for every clinical topic and to put each on 2"x3" index cards. Students must be selective with the information on the cards because these cards will be used during the clinical examination. Since only one card it permitted for every topic, students rewrite the cards several times during the semester. This strategy has ensured students' reading the material and facilitated the development of their ability to analyze the information. Students who have experienced this process shared valuable information, including:

- Their need to revise the cards as they learned more information and their thinking became more complex
- A perception of their improved ability to synthesize information
- A greater level of confidence in the examination

Students who were able to synthesize the clinical material were prepared for clinical and performed at a higher level on the examination. They admitted that they had no need to look at the cards during the examination. Some of their comments were, "Everything made sense," "I was never so prepared," and "What a creative way to test us."

32. How can faculty assist students with successful test taking on NCLEX and multiple choice exams?

The National Council Licensure Examination (NCLEX) format may have changed but the computerized adaptive testing (CAT) test plan has not. Students are fearful and experience much anxiety when taking multiple choice exams. Faculty can assist students by reducing their stress and anxiety. Students should be encouraged to practice stress reduction and relaxation exercises, such as listening to relaxation tapes, physical exercise, massage, or yoga. Anxiety can be decreased by focusing on three areas:

- Gaining information, developing skill, and decreasing unknowns
- Practicing basic strategies for successful test taking
- Advising students to monitor their time efficiently so as not to rush through the exam or run out of time

Nursing faculty should provide an exam review in a group or individually with students to review test performance. This is helpful in identifying students' test-taking problems. Students may have difficulty with comprehension of the content or may have a test-taking-personality that hinders their performance. Various test-taking personalities include:

- The Rusher, who is in a hurry to complete the exam
- The Turtle, who moves slowly through the exam, not leaving time at the end to finish the exam
- Others who may philosophize, use personal knowledge and insight, second-guess themselves, or too carefully scrutinize the question, "reading into the question"

Regardless of which of the above types characterizes the student, the approach may, in some cases, work well; more often, however, it may hinder the student's overall performance on an exam. To address this problem, refer the student to the college/university tutoring center, encourage students to join a study group, or encourage students to work with a counselor to address test-taking problems. The most beneficial time to identify students' test-taking problems is early in the course. As with other student problems, early intervention allows time for students to seek supportive assistance to remedy their performance on multiple choice exams.

An additional strategy for preparing students to take NCLEX is to take computer-based practice examinations that follow the NCLEX test plan and design. This practice will enhance familiarity with the format of the NCLEX exam, so that the student does not err due to unfamiliarity with the test format. The mechanics of answering questions on the NCLEX examination differ from other computer-based testing in several ways:

- Students cannot scroll back to review previous questions and answers.
- The stem of the question and distractors are displayed in a side-by-side format on the monitor.
- Moving forward to the next question submits the answer for the previous question.

Students who take the NCLEX exam without this knowledge beforehand can become confused and anxious at a time when they need to relax and concentrate on the questions.

Students about to graduate should be encouraged to develop a systematic plan of study in preparation for the NCLEX. NCLEX review courses are very beneficial for most students when preparing for the examination. Above all, students should be *discouraged* from relying solely on their basic nursing education program as the *only* method of preparation for NCLEX.

33. What are some basic rules for test-taking that enhance performance on multiple choice exams, including NCLEX?

The basic rules of test-taking include:
- Read the test question with an understanding of the parts (stem, correct answer, distractors).
- Read each question carefully; identify key words or phrases.
- Do not assume information that is not given.
- Eliminate answers that are obviously incorrect.
- Select responses that represent basic, idealistic nursing practice.
- Do not change answers without a *very* good reason (remind students that they cannot change answers on NCLEX).

34. The persistent concerns expressed by senior students are those of feeling unready to practice nursing and insecurity about independent clinical decisions making. How can I approach this issue?

Role transition to patient care management is filled with challenges and responsibilities that confront nursing students and new graduates. Students voice persistent concerns related to their socialization as novice nurses, making independent clinical decisions, and understanding the health care organization. Try the following strategies to assist students in these areas:

- Make sure that the curriculum addresses content related to the legal and ethical responsibilities of providing care, understanding the organization of various health care facilities, the role of professional nursing organizations, trends and economic issues related to patient care, and the utilization of nursing research in practice.
- Case studies, using case management with critical pathways, or a dialectic approach: student-precepted clinical experiences (near the end of the program) that enable students to work one-on-one with a registered nurse, facilitates role transition, the development of self-confidence, and socialization to the profession.

BIBLIOGRAPHY

1. Alfaro-LeFevre R: Critical Thinking in Nursing. Philadelphia, WB Saunders, 1998.
2. All AC, Havens RL: Cognitive/concept mapping: A teaching strategy for nursing. J Adv Nurs 25:1210-1219, 1997.
3. Beitz JM: Concept mapping: Navigating the learning process. Nurse Educator 23:35-41, 1998.
4. Billings DM, Halstead JA. Teaching Nursing: A Guide for Faculty. Philadelphia, WB Saunders, 1998.
5. Clark CM: Substance abuse among nursing students. Nurse Educator 24:16-19.
6. Foundation for Critical Thinking. Sonoma, CA, Sonoma State University, 1999. http://www.criticalthinking.org/University/default.html

7. Gary FA, Sigsby LM, Campbell D: Preparing for the 21st century: Diversity in nursing education, research, and practice. J Prof Nurs 14:272-279, 1998.
8. Haffer AG, Raingruber BJ: Discovering confidence in clinical reasoning and critical thinking development in baccalaureate nursing students. J Nurs Educ 37:61-70 , 1998.
9. Mahat G: Stress and coping: junior baccalaureate nursing students in clinical settings. Nurs Forum 33:11-19, 1998.
10. Musinski B: The educator as facilitator: a new kind of leadership. Nurs Forum 34:23-29, 1999.
11. Sides M, Korchek N: Nurse's Guide to Successful Test-Taking, 2nd ed. Philadelphia, JB Lippincott, 1994.
12. Strader M, Decker P: Role Transition to Patient Care Management. Norwalk, CT, Appleton & Lange, 1995.

15. STUDENTS WITH SPECIAL NEEDS

Linda J. Allan Pasto, MS, RN, and Geraldine Valencia-Go, PhD, RN

1. What is meant by a special needs student?

There are two types of special needs students:
- Students from disadvantaged (challenged) backgrounds who have the potential to succeed in a nursing program, but whose secondary educational experience has not provided the necessary foundation for college-level work
- Students who are academically qualified for a nursing program, but who have visual, hearing, mobility, learning, or mental disabilities, or a chronic illness such as diabetes or epilepsy which might impede progress in a nursing program

The term "disadvantaged" carries a negative, stigmatizing connotation; therefore, faculty are urged to use the term "challenged" when referring to a student's background.

2. What criteria are used to classify students as coming from a challenged background?

One or more of the following criteria are present for students from challenged backgrounds:
- Inadequate secondary education that did not prepare the student for college-level work
- Marginal secondary school records
- Inadequate financial resources, requiring the student to work to earn enough money to support himself or herself through college; working usually prohibits the student from taking advantage of available resources at the college or university
- Lack of appropriate role models and support systems for college attendance
- Has a primary language other than English, which creates a barrier to learning and interaction
- Student's community or neighborhood lacks adequate resources to support educational pursuits and professional development

3. How can faculty identify students from challenged backgrounds?

This is a difficult task at times. As faculty, we must be careful to avoid stereotyping the student and making the student feel "singled out." Schools whose mission is to provide equal access often have screening mechanisms in place to identify students from challenged backgrounds. However, any student who fits the above criteria should raise the index of suspicion in faculty and admissions counselors. Strategies that faculty can use to screen students' basic academic skills, social skills, and English language proficiency include:
- Assessment of student learning early in the course (quizzes, writing exercises)
- Standardized tests to assess learning style; critical thinking skills; math, reading, and verbal skills; social support; and self-esteem
- Peer support group with a faculty mentor
- Learn about students as individuals

4. What are the common issues that students from challenged backgrounds deal with and how can faculty help them?

Strategies for Addressing Issues in Students from Challenged Backgrounds

ISSUE	STRATEGY
Stigma, which often results in the student waiting until few or no alternatives are left to resolve problems	• Offer all resources and support services to all students to avoid singling out these students. • Create teaching-learning activities that incorporate the use of these services.
Lack of positive academic/professional role models	• Invite key members of local professional nursing organizations and/or professional nurses to mentor these students. • Encourage faculty to mentor these students.
Problems with speaking English and developing good writing skills	• Include short writing exercises and class presentations in your course. • Suggest movies to see and books to read to build language skills. • Encourage the student to speak English to family.
Inadequate time to study, since the student needs to work to support self or family	• Assist students to obtain part-time jobs as research assistants with faculty who have funded studies (this enables students to perform work that is scholarly in nature, e.g., literature searches, data collection, data entry; such work helps to build academic skills). • Help students seek scholarships for health professions students or refer students to a financial aid counselor.
Lack of trust in an unfamiliar social and academic system (no one speaks student's primary language, understands his or her customs, or acknowledges his or her concerns and issues)	• Persons who have initial contact with new students must have excellent interpersonal skills and a thorough knowledge of the institution's resources. This person (or someone else) should be a designated ombudsman for students.
Lack of appropriate role models in their home (often results in a lack of familial support)	• Provide orientation for students and parents on the same day. Parents unable to attend could be given a video (in their primary language) or invited back to the institution for a rescheduled orientation. • Parents can also be invited to attend a class or laboratory where students are learning psycho-motor skills. (This strategy assumes that the student has parents who are present in the home, are interested in the student's success, speak English, and have the resources to travel to campus or watch a video at home.)

5. How can the institution foster a sense of community among students from challenged backgrounds?

Begin on day one, when students are oriented to the school. If the college or university does not have an orientation program, the nursing program could develop its own orientation for new students. Many orientation programs are directed at first-time, full-time freshmen. However, it behooves the school to offer orientation to transfer students also. A well-structured orientation program smooths the student's transition to the new environment and experiences.

Provide opportunities for students to meet other students and become involved in student organizations. Depending upon the resources of your institution, you may be able to develop a special program to mainstream these students. Examples of special programs include a multicultural day that celebrates diversity (students, faculty, and administrators should collaborate to plan the activities) and/or a students' organization day during which all student organizations share their goals and completed projects. Other strategies include inviting minority speakers from local health care facilities or professional organizations, recruiting minority faculty and staff, and creating an advisory committee to help in planning effective strategies to address the needs of students from challenged backgrounds.

6. Aside from coming from a challenged background, what are some other common special needs that nursing students present with?

Other common special needs include learning disabilities, attention deficit disorder, physical challenges such as hearing and sight deficits, and mobility deficits.

7. Which special needs students should be admitted to a nursing program?

Many students who are academically qualified, but disabled, could potentially complete the nursing program. An academically qualified student with learning or physical disabilities should be viewed as having the potential to become a registered nurse, and alternative paths for helping the student achieve his or her goals should be examined. Some students, however, will have learning or physical disabilities that are too restrictive to meet minimal requirements for nursing, and should be counseled into other majors that are aligned with their interests.

Students from challenged backgrounds who demonstrate academic potential can also be admitted to the nursing program, provided there are adequate resources available at the college or university to address their needs. While it is important to recognize students' potential, it is equally important to provide adequate support services or reasonable accommodations for special needs students. To do otherwise sets the student up for failure, a situation to be avoided at all costs.

8. What is the Americans with Disabilities Act?

The Americans with Disabilities Act is one of two laws that affect individuals with disabilities. The other is the Rehabilitation Act of 1973, Section 504. The Rehabilitation Act stipulates that any institution that receives federal funds cannot discriminate against students with disabilities and must make appropriate adjustments to its policies and procedures to allow such students to fully participate in its programs. The law does not require colleges and universities to alter the content of programs offered or the skills and knowledge required of the graduates of the program. The ADA states that no institution may discriminate on the basis of disability. It extends antidiscrimination laws to employment, housing, architectural accessibility, professional licensing, and education. Post-secondary education must provide reasonable accommodations, which may include testing adjustments, adjustments to academic requirements, tape recording, auxiliary aids, and services.

9. How do the Rehabilitation Act of 1973 and the Americans with Disabilities Act of 1990 affect my teaching?

By law, reasonable accommodations must be provided if the college or university has adequate documentation of the disability and if the student's disability allows him or her protection under the ADA. These accommodations may be accessible through an office within the educational institution or the nursing department. Nursing faculty need to work with the college disabilities coordinator to ensure that they are acting within the law.

Current legal action (case law) continues to define the way in which the courts interpret who is protected by the law and what accommodations are reasonable. If a student has already been evaluated and a disability documented, the faculty member needs to work with the plan that has been established for this individual. If faculty suspect that a student has a disability, they need to encourage the student to obtain an evaluation so that accommodations can be provided as indicated.

Nursing programs should encourage disclosure of special needs to allow accommodations to be provided at the beginning of a student's academic career. Students may be reluctant to approach a faculty member or disclose this information based on previous negative experiences. They may have experienced low self-esteem and subsequently will require extra support to ensure success for the student.

10. What is a reasonable accommodation?

Usually, it is easier to define what *is not* reasonable, which, logically, allows you to assume that if the accommodation does not fall within these parameters, it probably *is* reasonable. An *unreasonable* accommodation:

- Presents a direct threat to the heath and safety of others
- Causes a substantial change in the curriculum or in the way services are provided
- Causes an undue financial or administrative burden

Reasonable accommodations can include testing adjustments, such as extra time for testing, a separate area for taking tests, a reader for tests, and alternative methods of assessment that are sensitive to the student's special needs. Adjustments to academic requirements could involve course substitution, changes in the length of time allowed for completion of degree requirements, and adaptations in the way a course is taught. Also included might be permission to tape record in class as well as auxiliary aids and services, such as extended time for assignment and test completion, taped or oral examinations, large print exams and answer sheets, readers, scribes, interpreters, taped texts as well as classroom equipment adaptation. Students can be accommodated with arrangements such as videotaped lectures and access to class notes.

11. Are students with disabilities required to report their disability?

No. A student only needs to disclose this information if he or she requests accommodations. Students should feel that their information will be treated with respect and support. A statement outlining students' rights at the institution, as well as the process to obtain assistance, should be included in student handbooks and college catalogs. Faculty should include a statement in the course syllabus which encourages students with special needs to make their needs known to the student disabilities coordinator.

12. What teaching methods would be most effective for students with special needs?

The answer to this, of course, depends upon what the student's needs are. Specific methods for some of the more common disabilities will be covered later in the chapter. Some general approaches that could be implemented include:

- The use of multimodal teaching approaches, for example, music, color, movement, and oral participation

- Clear and structured expectations for a course, clinical, seminar, and lab which provide as much detail as possible (of course, you would expect to provide this for all students in your class!)
- A team planning conference to coordinate approaches to the student's learning; include the college's disabilities coordinator
- Consultation with the student to determine types of accommodations that have already been used successfully
- An "approachable" demeanor, since students often attribute their success to faculty who are willing to help meet their needs
- Flexibility in program and course requirements; discuss possible options proactively rather than in response to a request
- Provide instruction in time management, note taking, test taking, and organizational skills early in the program
- Counsel students to consider completing requirements over a longer period of time (within reason) to increase chances of success
- Ensure that lecture is not the primary mode of information transmission; many students with special needs will benefit from different teaching methods

13. What is the most common disability reported by nursing programs?

Learning disabilities. Twenty-five percent of all students reporting a disability indicate a learning disability. This number is expected to increase because 50% of learning disabled high school students are expected to seek a college education.

14. What is a learning disability?

One of the most widely accepted definitions is from the Learning Disabilities Association. This organization offers the following definition:

"…a chronic condition of presumed neurological origin which selectively interferes with the development, integration and/or demonstration of verbal and nonverbal abilities. Specific learning disabilities exist as a distinct handicapping condition in the presence of average to superior intelligence, adequate sensory and motor systems, and adequate learning opportunities. The condition varies in its manifestations and in the degree of severity throughout life. The condition can affect self-esteem, education, vocation, socialization, and daily living activities."

15. How is a learning disability identified?

The student may voluntarily report a learning difficulty that has been previously diagnosed. Clues that a student might have a learning disability include:

- A discrepancy between what the student can verbally report and what he or she produces in a testing format, i.e., the student can explain information that he or she was unable to produce in a written mode
- The ability to process information when he or she reads something, but difficulty understanding what is presented orally in class
- Difficulty with at least one mode of learning, but one mode of learning that works well

Once a discrepancy in the student's performance has been noted, the student should be evaluated so that the most effective approaches can be utilized. If screening is done by your institution prior to admission, some of these discrepancies may be detected and further assessment done at that time.

Keep in mind that some students avoid disclosure based on previous negative experiences. Students may feel that their disability would prevent successful progress through the nursing program. They should be counseled on their options and rights under the law.

16. What specific characteristics will I be most likely to note in the learning disabled student?

Students with deficient reading skills may demonstrate a slower than normal reading rate and poor comprehension and retention of what is read. They may complain about the heavy reading load or how far behind they are in their reading. New vocabulary may be difficult. Students with deficient reading skills may express difficulty with the ability to identify themes or to highlight important points in their reading. Writing difficulties may also present and are manifested as poor sentence structure, spelling errors, the inability to correctly copy from a book or blackboard, slower than normal writing skills, and poor penmanship.

Students with deficient oral language and processing skills often demonstrate the following characteristics:
- An inability to concentrate on and comprehend oral language
- Difficulty formulating and orally expressing ideas
- Evidence of better written expression than oral expression
- Difficulty pronouncing and speaking grammatically correct English

Because much of a student's learning is presented in an oral mode, language and language processing skills are an important area to evaluate early in order to prevent the student from getting too far behind.

Students with math disabilities demonstrate incomplete mastery of basic mathematic facts, reversal of numbers, confusion of operational symbols, the inability to copy problems correctly, and reasoning difficulties. Mathematic computation, application, and abstract problems pose the most difficulty.

Study and social skills present many challenges to the learning-disabled college student. Typical of these difficulties are time management difficulties, difficulties following oral and written directions, and the lack of organizational skills. Socially, the student may have difficulty interpreting verbal and nonverbal messages with peers, faculty, and clients.

17. How can I best help a learning disabled student to learn?

Use a variety of teaching techniques to facilitate understanding of the information presented. If you suspect that a student has a learning disability, refer the student to the college or university's disabilities coordinator. Faculty development workshops will assist faculty to identify problems early and to provide reasonable accommodations, if indicated.

18. What specific accommodations would be considered "reasonable" for a student with a learning disability?

Each disability student's situation must be evaluated individually. This is certainly one case where the "one size fits all" rule does not apply. Generally speaking, the following accommodations might be beneficial and reasonable for students with learning disabilities:
- Access to taped textbooks
- Access to instructor notes
- Extended deadlines for papers and projects
- Untimed tests or extra time for testing
- Review of previously covered material at the beginning of each class
- Summary of key points at the end of each class
- Emphasis on new vocabulary or terms
- Questioning to monitor understanding
- Assignments provided in both written and oral modes
- Clear and early discussion of all expectations provided in written and oral modes
- The use of tape recorders during class
- Textbooks with ancillary student learning aids (study guides, computer-assisted instruction)

• An alternative format for the completion of papers or projects
• Alternative testing modes and supplemental test aids (oral tests, use of computers, calculators, portfolio assessment)

Students should be encouraged to use the following strategies to compensate for their disabilities:

• Participate in a study group
• Write questions during class about confusing material, to be reviewed with faculty after class
• Use all available learning resources available at the college or university, i.e., computer-assisted instruction, videotapes related to course content, tutoring
• Begin assignments early to allow for the additional time needed to complete the work

19. What if the learning disabled student has difficulty with math skills and struggles to calculate medication dosages correctly?

This is an interesting and provocative question! In a hypothetical situation, students' drug calculation skills can be evaluated in any of several ways. If the student struggles with pencil and paper tests, try to allow extra time for testing or remove all time limits. If the student is unsuccessful with a pencil and paper test, consider setting up a "challenge" in the lab, using actual equipment. A drug calculation problem can be set up using syringes, medicine cups, and a supply of the "drug," with actual calculations to be performed by the student. Allowing students to manipulate the equipment may enable their ability to calculate the dose correctly. Sometimes students may be able to correctly calculate in the clinical setting where they can explain the process to the clinical instructor. A student may also be able to demonstrate performance with a computer simulation. The important point to remember is: If a student is struggling with a particular evaluation mode, use an alternative testing mode to provide an opportunity for the student to demonstrate his or her knowledge. *If the student still cannot demonstrate correct performance after having the opportunity to test using alternative methods, then he or she may not be able to overcome the deficit to the degree that is needed to succeed.*

20. What is attention deficit disorder (ADD)?

ADD is a neurobiological disorder characterized by behaviors that impair a person's ability to function effectively in his or her environment. The disorder is estimated to occur in 3–5% of the United States population. It is more frequently diagnosed in males and underdiagnosed in females. Females are more likely to be diagnosed after childhood, often showing up in college, and more specifically, in nursing programs. Undiagnosed ADD can contribute to poor student performance.

21. What behaviors would I expect to see in a student with ADD?

• Has difficulty paying attention in the classroom
• Gets lower than average grades
• Lacks motivation
• Procrastinates on completion of assignments (but when completed, may be very well done)
• Has difficulty following directions, even when very specific
• Forgets important appointments and commitments
• Lacks a system for organizing notes and materials
• Cannot recall data that require memorization
• Experiences difficulty in delaying gratification, i.e., needs attention/answers *now*
• Changes jobs or careers frequently

• Has difficulty with interpersonal communications
• Demonstrates above-average creativity
• Exhibits spontaneity
• Focuses intensely on activities of interest
• Has a wide field of vision

22. How can I help a student with ADD?

Refer the student with possible undiagnosed ADD to the learning disabilities specialist at your college or university. Emphasize to the student the importance of establishing a diagnosis through a health care provider rather than by self-assessment. Documentation of any disability is required to initiate the formal academic accommodation.

A health care provider will rule out other neurological or psychological conditions and may be able to prescribe medications to mitigate symptoms. A concurrent referral may be needed for supportive counseling to address the often coexisting problems of anxiety, depression, and/or substance abuse. A referral to career counseling may be necessary for the student who is unable to achieve success despite appropriate academic accommodations.

23. What specific techniques will help the student with ADD in both the classroom and clinical setting?

Although the following tips can be applied to any student to enhance learning, for the student with ADD, these strategies can mean the difference between success and failure:

• Establish clear standards for student performance and expect achievement of normal course requirements.
• Develop a behavioral contract with the student: set goals with time lines both in the classroom and clinical setting
• Be receptive to innovative, creative approaches that may be used by students to accomplish their educational and clinical goals.
• Establish assignment deadlines, encourage structure in study techniques, and expect accountability.
• Recognize and reward success in classroom and clinical settings.
• Encourage the student to use color in note-taking and studying, since ADD individuals are visually oriented.
• Use multimodal learning techniques (give assignments in writing and orally, use visual aids that incorporate color, use physical movements during class).
• Teach memory aids and outlining.
• Repeat, Repeat, Repeat!!
• Develop tests that measure knowledge, not attention span.
• Be available to meet with student to monitor progress, and provide feedback and support (be aware that the student may have had negative experiences in the education system and, therefore, you may need to initiate meetings).
• Consider eliminating time restraints for tests and/or assignments, initially.
• Help the student break tasks or assignments into smaller manageable units.

24. What is the best approach for the students with special physical needs?

First, encourage the student to determine if the disability is so limiting that he or she may not be employable as a nurse. A student should be afforded career counseling to explore possibilities congruent with his or her special physical need(s). If it is determined that the student has the potential to complete the nursing program and gain employment as a registered nurse, then reasonable accommodations must be provided as required.

Assistive devices may enable students to function effectively in the clinical setting. For a student with a hearing loss, an amplified stethoscope can be effective for auscultation. Keep in mind, though, that students need to be able to hear equipment alarms unless visual alternatives are available. A visually impaired student may need large print texts, assignment sheets, and other course materials. However, the student needs to be able to read common measures, such as sphygmomanometer dials, scales, thermometers, monitor screens, and gauges with the use of assistive devices. A student with mobility or limb deficits may require a comparable but safe client assignment to meet clinical objectives. Not every student needs to get a 300-pound stroke patient out of bed for the first time! Reasonable accommodations include the use of assistive devices and alternative assignments. However, the bottom line is that all students need to meet minimum safety performance standards for patient care.

25. What should I do if I believe that the student's disability will impede practice as a registered nurse?

Encourage the student need to look at the disability realistically to evaluate whether he or she would ever be employable as a registered nurse. A general discussion with other faculty, local employers, and career counselors may uncover possibilities that the student had not considered. Creative approaches to clinical assignments may allow disabled students to meet the same objectives as nondisabled students, just in different ways. When it becomes apparent that the student's disability is greater than first believed, then it might be wise to refer the student to career counseling.

When you are concerned about a student's progress, DOCUMENT! Anecdotal notes and clinical evaluations can be used to validate your concerns about a student's ability to achieve clinical objectives and ultimately attain employment as a registered nurse. Remember, though, that anecdotal notes can be subpoenaed and should provide evidence that the student had ample and varied opportunities to demonstrate learning. Moreover, anecdotal notes and clinical evaluations should document unsafe behaviors and the circumstances in which the behaviors occurred. Faculty are advised, however, that if anecdotal notes are kept, they should be kept on all students, and should reflect strengths as well as weaknesses for all students. Anecdotal notes are part of the student record and, as such, are protected by the Buckley Amendment; therefore, the student has the right to examine them and respond to inaccuracies. (For more information on this topic, refer to the chapter, "Legal and Ethical Issues.")

26. How can faculty foster a positive learning environment for all special needs students?

The most critical aspects in fostering a positive learning environment are trust and openness, where expectations and standards are made clear at the beginning of every course. Consider establishing a written contract with the student. Such a contract establishes the context of the teaching-learning process and facilitates awareness and understanding of the collaboration and/or accommodations that are needed in all settings. Other valuable strategies include:

- Maintain the same standards for all students.
- Do not accept substandard work from students.
- Address unacceptable behavior in a timely manner; discuss with the student his or her plans to modify the behavior.
- Answer all questions about classroom material; adopt the motto: "There are no stupid questions".
- Insist that students respect other's opinions.
- Encourage students to share their experiences; students often learn vicariously from each other.
- Provide equal opportunities for all students to speak during class.

- Recognize individual and group contributions.
- Provide credit whenever and wherever appropriate.
- Accentuate the positive in a negative situation, but remember to address the negative.
- Be willing to validate information and admit errors; students do not expect faculty to be walking encyclopedias, and they can readily tell when faculty don't know the answers; besides, admitting an error or lack of knowledge about something sets a positive example for students to do the same.
- Remember that alternative does not mean less than.
- Document behaviors, accommodations, and counseling provided, resources accessed, and student interactions.
- Be creative in approaching the needs of students.
- Expect a great deal and help students develop their potential.
- Use humor both in teaching and in working with students.
- Remember that some students just can't be successful, no matter how much you and they want success.
- Consider counseling students who have failed courses, or are significantly struggling, to take alternative routes to a nursing career.
- Praise, approve, support, and nourish!

BIBLIOGRAPHY

1. Campbell AR, Davis SM: Faculty commitment: retaining minority students in majority institutions. J Nurs Educ 35:298-303, 1996.
2. Colon EJ: Identification, accommodation, and success of students with learning disabilities in nursing education programs. J Nurs Educ 36:372-377, 1997.
3. Dowell MA: Issues in recruitment and retention of minority nursing students. J Nurs Educ 35:293-297, 1996.
4. Eliason M: Nursing students with learning disabilities: appropriate accommodations. J Nurs Ed 21:375-376, 1992.
5. Heyward S: Disability and Higher Education: Guidance for Section 504 and ADA Compliance. Horsham, PA, LRP Publications, 1998.
6. Jarrow J: Title by Title: The ADA's Impact on Post-Secondary Education. Columbus, OH, Association on Higher Education and Disability, 1992.
7. Letzia M: Issues in the post-secondary education of learning-disabled nursing students. Nurse Ed 20:18-22, 1995.
8. Maglivy JK, Mitchell AC: Education of nursing students with special needs. J Nurs Ed 34:31-6, 1995.
9. Vance C, Olson RK: The Mentor Connection in Nursing. New York, Springer, 1998.
10. Weber MC: Disability discrimination in higher education. J College Univ Law 26: 351-77, 1999.

16. STUDENT EVALUATION

Linda J. Scheetz, EdD, RN, CS, CEN

1. What does evaluation really mean?

The process of evaluation implies decision making about the student's ability to perform in the classroom as well as in the clinical setting. An important component of the evaluation process is the measurement of the student's ability. Measurement and evaluation go hand-in-hand. Measuring ability (through the use of tests, observation, written assignments, and so on) precedes the evaluation component, that is, the actual decision making about whether the student passes or fails. Therefore, evaluation is a deliberate, rational, systematic process based upon measurement principles.

2. Why is student evaluation an issue in nursing education?

Student evaluation is a big issue in education, especially nursing education, because the outcome of the educational process is preparation for professional practice. Therefore, faculty are the gatekeepers to the profession. As such, they decide who meets the standards for professional practice and who does not. This gatekeeping responsibility should not be taken lightly or performed in an arbitrary manner. Faculty should use the most valid and reliable methods available to them to evaluate students.

3. How do I determine the best way to evaluate students?

The first step in evaluating students is knowing what the outcomes of the course or particular activity are. What do you want students to know or do at the completion of the course or activity? Once you have identified the outcomes, you will be able to identify one or more possible ways to measure the achievement of the outcomes. Try to vary your methods of evaluation within a course. For example, you might want to administer several exams and quizzes, and perhaps include a written assignment or two. Some students perform best on exams; other students are better at writing papers. Students who were educated in other countries are often not familiar with multiple-choice questions and, therefore, are better able to demonstrate their knowledge with essay questions or a written assignment. A variety of evaluation methods accommodate different student styles and provide a more comprehensive view of actual learning than using just one method of evaluation.

4. Most of the testing done in our nursing program relates to the cognitive domain. Is this adequate?

Faculty do have a tendency to limit paper and pencil testing to measure the cognitive domain. Evaluation of the psychomotor domain occurs in the clinical setting and, in some instances, in the nursing laboratory. The affective domain is the domain that is often under-evaluated. Because all nursing programs aspire to produce competent entry-level practitioners, it behooves nursing faculty to evaluate students in the affective domain as well as in the cognitive and psychomotor domains. Affective domain competencies can be measured with paper-and-pencil testing and observation of performance in the clinical setting.

5. How do I go about constructing a test?

Begin with a test blueprint. Just as an architect's blueprint guides the construction of a building, a teacher's test blueprint guides the construction of a test. The test blueprint should be a matrix that includes the following:

- Unit objectives (outcomes) and content
- Cognitive level (knowledge, comprehension, application, analysis, evaluation, synthesis)

You might also include steps of the nursing process (assessment, analysis, planning, implementation, evaluation) in your blueprint, although it is difficult to envision a 3-dimensional matrix. However, including questions at the application and analysis levels that focus on various steps of the nursing process is important if your goal is to test critical thinking.

Test Blueprint for One Unit of a Physical Assessment Course

OBJECTIVE	COGNITIVE LEVEL	NO. OF QUESTIONS
Objective: Describe normal physical assessment findings of the cardiovascular system.	knowledge	2
	comprehension	2
	application	4
	analysis	3
Content: Heart and peripheral vascular system		
Objective: Describe information the nurse collects when taking a patient history relative to the cardiovascular system.	knowledge	2
	comprehension	2
	application	4
	analysis	2
Content: Chief complaint, medications, allergies, past medical history, psychosocial history, health maintenance activities, diet, exercise, leisure activities		
Objective: Differentiate normal and abnormal findings relative to the cardiovascular system.	knowledge	4
	comprehension	4
	application	6
	analysis	5
Content: Inspection, auscultation, percussion, palpation of heart and peripheral vascular system		
	Total # questions	40

Next, determine what types of questions you will include (multiple choice, essay, matching, true-false, fill-in-the blank). Multiple choice and essay questions are most commonly used on nursing tests since they lend themselves to measuring various levels of the cognitive and affective domains. On the other hand, matching, true-false, and fill-in-the-blank questions generally measure only the first two levels of the cognitive domain; therefore, their usefulness is limited. Third, determine the length of the test (how many questions you want to include). The number of questions will depend on the time available for students to complete the test. Multiple choice questions usually require 60-90 seconds each to complete. Essay questions require time for collecting thoughts, formulating an outline, and actually writing the response.

Test construction is time-consuming but well worth the effort. So, allow plenty of time, roll up your sleeves, and get started. This is one of those tasks that you will need to set aside a large block of time to accomplish.

6. What type of test questions are best to use on a paper-and-pencil test?

The "best" type of question will be determined by the purpose of the test and what you intend to measure. Are you developing a major exam or a 10-minute quiz? The table below offers a comparison of various types of test questions. Depending upon the purpose and scope of the test, you may want to select just one type of question or combine types of questions.

Advantages and Disadvantages of Various Types of Test Questions

TYPE OF QUESTION	ADVANTAGES	DISADVANTAGES
Multiple choice	Measures all cognitive and affective domain levels; easy to correct	Time-consuming to develop
Essay (complex)	Easy to develop; measures higher cognitive and affective domain levels	Time-consuming to correct; grading often lacks consistency
True-false	Easy to correct	Measures lowest level (knowledge) of cognitive domain; difficult to develop questions with absolute answers
Matching	Easy to construct; easy to correct	Measures lowest level (knowledge) of cognitive domain
Completion (fill-in-the-blanks)	Easy to correct	Difficult to measure higher cognitive and affective domain levels; blanks may have different interpretations by different students (questions lack validity)
Short-answer essay	Easy to contruct	May be time-consuming to correct; grading often lacks consistency

7. What is an item analysis and why should I perform it?

An item analysis is an analysis of an exam that is performed after students have completed the exam. The item analysis is performed by analyzing students' responses to test items. Item analysis measures the difficulty level of each question and the test as a whole, as well as the discriminatory ability of each question. (Discriminatory ability is the ability of the test question to distinguish between those students who know the correct answer and those who do not know.) Once you have developed a test, be sure to conduct an item analysis after the test has been given. An item analysis serves several purposes:

- Provides evidence of the difficulty level of the test
- Identifies how well students understand selected content
- Distinguishes those students who know the answers from those who do not

The item analysis usually includes measures of central tendency, such as the range of test scores, mean score, median score, mode, and standard deviation. While it is possible to perform an item analysis manually, optical scanners perform the analysis for each question as the exam is being graded.

The results of the item analysis can be used as follows:

- Adjust test scores, if indicated. (Not all test questions are well-constructed; if a question is poorly constructed, the item analysis will provide evidence of this. Eliminate the question and recalculate the test scores.)
- Modify questions for future use. (Change distractors; re-word questions to improve their validity).
- Identify course content that needs additional emphasis.

Pearl: Keep quizzes and tests secure, i.e., do not allow students to copy or keep the test questions. You never know when you might want to re-use them.

Pearl: Once you have refined test questions and adjusted the difficulty level of your test so that you have a "really good test," keep it secure and use it again! Because good test questions evolve over time, based on modification from item analyses, it behooves faculty to save and re-use "good" test questions.

8. Should I be using computer-based testing?

Recognize that computers are a medium to accomplish the task, just as paper-and-pencil tests are. There is no mystery about using computers to test students. Commercially prepared computer examinations are available; most have reliability and validity data available, which is a plus. Software is available that enables faculty to construct their own computer-based tests. Many computer-assisted instruction programs include a test at the end of the teaching material so that students can self-test. The use of computer-based testing offers the following advantages:

- Student self-evaluation (with computer-assisted instruction)
- Ease of administration (students log onto the network or insert the disk)
- Ease of grading (commercially prepared test software grades the exam and sometimes even includes a grade book)
- Enhanced test security (it is more difficult for students to cheat, since handwritten answers are not available for copying)
- Familiarizes the student with computer-based testing, which might allay anxiety about the mechanics of taking NCLEX
- Generates data that can be used for curriculum and/or course evaluation (many commercially prepared tests generate aggregate as well as individual data)

9. What about using the test banks provided by textbook publishers?

Test banks are usually developed to be used with specific textbooks. For example, a publisher publishes a medical-surgical nursing textbook, then contracts with one or more authors to develop a test bank to accompany that book. Test banks that are designed to be used with designated textbooks may be useful, especially for novice faculty who have never developed test questions. One limitation of commercially prepared test banks is that they frequently test the lower levels of the cognitive domain. A second limitation is that they are often very focused on the accompanying textbook. Therefore, if you intend to test application and analysis of both the cognitive and affective domains, the usefulness of these questions is limited.

As with the construction of any test, plan ahead, allowing plenty of time to review questions that are included in the test bank. You may choose to use them verbatim or modify them.

10. I have heard that multiple-choice questions should be kept "simple." What does that mean?

The matter of simplicity relates to two issues: the domain level of the question and the mechanics of writing the question. First, the domain issue. Questions written at the lower levels of the cognitive domain tend to be more straightforward, since they measure only the skills of recall, recognition, etc. Questions that measure higher levels of the cognitive domain, such as application and analysis, require more information in the stem of the question. With application and analysis questions, students are asked to consider a patient situation, analyze relationships among data, and/or apply the information in a hypothetical situation. Therefore, when considering the issue of simplicity as it relates to different domains, recognize that questions which measure application and analysis will not be as "simple" (i.e., straightforward) as those that measure knowledge and comprehension. However, there are valid reasons for measuring the application and analysis domains, so write these questions carefully and include them on your test. *Pearl: You might find it helpful to ask a faculty colleague to a critique your questions, especially if you are a novice at writing test questions.*

Second, the mechanics of writing the question. Let's consider this issue as it relates to the stem, the correct answer, and the distractors of a multiple-choice question. It is a good idea *not* to include a lot of extraneous information in the stem of the question. While you will want to evaluate the student's ability to analyze relationships and select relevant data, too much unrelated information in the stem is confusing and adds no value to the test. As for the correct answer and distractors (incorrect answer choices), keep them simple, too.

Using distractors that list several possible answers and then require students to select combinations of the possibilities (sometimes referred to as "multiple-multiple choice") are confusing and do not add value to the measurement process. Contrary to the beliefs of some faculty, multiple-multiple choice questions do not discriminate any better between the strong and weak student than do simple multiple-choice questions.

To answer the question about simplicity, keep the following in mind:
• Avoid including extraneous information in the stem of the question.
• Keep the reading level and vocabulary of the questions appropriate for the level of the students.
• Use correct grammar and punctuation.
• Avoid using correct answers and distractors that include the following:
    • all of the above
    • none of the above
    • combinations of the above (e.g., A, C, D)

11. What is the best way to approach the grading of short answer and essay questions?

Short answer and longer essay questions do not pose the forced-choice response that multiple-choice questions pose. Therefore, students should be allowed to express creativity when proposing answers, provided there is adequate rationale for the answer. Have a general idea about the answer you are seeking, keeping in mind that students may propose correct answers that you had not thought of. If your question is very focused, thus limiting the possible range of answers, make a note of the answer that you consider correct. Establishing some reference points is important to do *before* you begin grading the tests, since doing so will improve the consistency of your grading.

Some faculty find it helpful to read all of the students' answers to a given question before grading any of the answers to get a sense of the range of answers. Then, go back and reread the tests, writing comments and adding/deducting points for the answers. It is also helpful to cover students' names to avoid the possibility of bias when reading answers.

The goal with short answer/essay questions is to stimulate students' creativity and critical thinking skills. Therefore, keep an open mind when considering the answers and maintain consistency when assigning grades.

12. What about using written assignments to measure students' achievement?

Written assignments provide a valuable method of evaluating students' achievement, while helping students to integrate content. Refer to the chapter, "Teaching Strategy: Written Assignments," for more about this topic.

13. What are some measurement issues that I should be concerned about?

Validity and reliability are issues that often plague faculty when evaluating students. Validity means that the instrument (test, clinical evaluation scale, etc.) measures what it was intended to measure. Reliability means that the instrument measures accurately and consistently.

Types of Reliability

TYPE OF RELIABILITY	DEFINITION	EXAMPLE
Interrater	Degree to which different raters (or faculty) arrive at the same conclusion (grade) for a given student when using the same instrument to measure performance simultaneously	Two faculty evaluate one student simultaneously using the same clinical evaluation instrument. The "closeness" of their rating is an estimate of interrater reliability.
Intrarater	Degree of consistency with which one faculty measures the same responses on different occasions	Faculty A grades student Z's answers to essay questions on day 1, again on day 8, and again on day 15. The degree of agreement between the scores is the intrarater reliability.
Test-retest	Degree to which a test measures consistently and accurately over time	A drug calculation test is used at the beginning of each semester. The degree to which the test accurately and consistently measures students' abilities to calculate drug dosages over time is test-retest reliability.
Internal consistency	Degree to which items on a test or clinical evaluation instrument measure the same concept	A medical-surgical course unit test has questions relating to the steps of the nursing process. Internal consistency is the degree to which test items relate to each of the concepts measures (e.g., assessment, analysis, planning, intervention, evaluation).[4]

Reliability estimates are correlation coefficients, ranging from 0 to 1.00, with 1.00 representing perfect reliability. Most measurement instruments fall somewhere in between. The higher the estimate, the better the instrument or test.

Unlike item difficulty and index of discrimination, reliability estimates are not determined by item analysis of a given test. Furthermore, determining these characteristics is time-consuming and difficult if faculty have not had formal instruction and practical experience with statistical analysis. Therefore, it is not common practice for faculty to determine the various types of reliability of course exams.

Given the significance of all evaluation measures used in nursing education, and the fact that students' futures are determined by these evaluations, one can easily understand why measurement and evaluation are such a big issue.

Evaluation of students' performance in the clinical setting is more difficult than paper-and-pencil evaluation in the classroom, since there is greater room for subjectivity in the process. Given the relative significance of clinical evaluations, it is imperative that faculty estimate the validity and reliability of all clinical evaluation instruments, since clinical evaluation is generally an all-or-nothing experience (students either pass or do not pass). Moreover, failure in clinical often results in failure of the entire course, regardless of grades on exams and written work.

From a legal perspective, the use of measurement instruments without evidence of acceptable validity and reliability could spell trouble for faculty, particularly if the student's career is brought to a standstill because of a course or clinical failure.

14. Everyone in our department uses a different clinical evaluation measure. Is this a problem?

It could be. Inherent in "good" evaluation is the use of "good" measurement instruments. By "good," we mean instruments that have acceptable validity and reliability. Moreover, measurement instruments, including tests and clinical evaluation instruments, should be sensitive enough to distinguish those who "know" from those who "don't know." This can be a tall order, considering that faculty often design tests and clinical evaluation instruments in haste with little knowledge of measurement principles. Kind of scary, huh?

One important aspect of clinical evaluation often overlooked by faculty is the *evolution of clinical competence* as the student progresses through the nursing program. In many nursing programs, faculty design their own clinical evaluation instruments, all of which are course specific. As such, there are few commonalities among instruments, and therefore, little ability to track students' development of clinical competence across the curriculum.

15. What are some issues with the construction of clinical evaluation instruments?

Validity and reliability. Validity is the first concern. Without validity, reliability is unimportant. Often, when faculty develop their own course-specific clinical evaluation instruments, they end up with instruments that do not measure the entire domain of behaviors included in the course (and performed in the clinical setting). Faculty, as a group, should define what they mean by clinical competence. Once that is done, elements of the definition should appear in the clinical objectives and clinical evaluation instrument for each course. However, such a process rarely occurs. More likely, each faculty member decides what is important to measure in the clinical setting used for his/her course. Some faculty focus on psychomotor skills, whereas others zero in on cognitive skills, often expressing items in ways that are not measurable, yielding little meaningful information regarding the clinical competence of the student.

Once valid items representing the domain of clinical competence and clinical objectives have been identified for the course, the next challenge faced by faculty is developing instruments that are reliable. Instruments should be as free from measurement error and bias as possible. Your goal is to measure the same clinical behaviors accurately and consistently over time in all students enrolled in the course. Developing a valid instrument to do so can take a year or more.

16. Is there a clinical evaluation instrument that has acceptable reliability and validity?

Yes. The Clinical Competence Rating Scale (CCRS),[2] developed in 1988, has acceptable reliability and validity (see Appendix A). The conceptual definition of clinical competence from which the CCRS items were derived encompasses the student's ability to engage in problem solving, apply theory to practice, and perform psychomotor skills. The unique feature of the CCRS is its applicability across the undergraduate nursing curriculum. The instrument can be used in all nursing content areas (e.g., medical-surgical, pediatrics, maternity, psych-mental health, community health). Therefore, faculty can track the development of clinical competence in students as they progress through the curriculum. Likewise, areas of performance difficulty are easy to detect.

Appendix A
Clinical Competence Rating Scale

CLINICAL COMPETENCE RATING SCALE (CCRS)
DEFINITION OF THE RATING SCALE LABELS*

Label Name and Performance According to Accepted Standards of Performance and Quality of Assistance Required

Independent	Safe, accurate Appropriate affect each time Desired outcome each time	Proficient, coordinated, confident Occasional expenditure of excess energy	None
Supervised	Safe, accurate Appropriate affect each time Desired outcome each time	Efficient, coordinated Some expenditure of excess energy Task completed within a reasonable time	Occasional supporting cues needed
Assisted	Safe, accurate Affect appropriate most of the time Desired outcome most of the time	Skilled in parts of the behavior Inefficient and uncoordinated Excess energy expended to accomplish task Requires delayed time to complete task	Supportive cues Occasional physical cues needed Frequent verbal cues needed
Marginal	Safe, but not alone Desired outcome some of the time Affect appropriate occasionally	Unskilled, inefficient Considerable expenditure of excess energy Requires prolonged time to complete task	Continuous verbal and physical cues needed
Dependent	Unsafe Unable to demonstrate behavior	Lacks confidence Uncoordinated, inefficient	Continuous verbal and physical cues needed

Not applicable
Not observed

Scoring. To assign a numerical grade for clinical performance, the following values may be used:

Independent (I)	5
Supervised (S)	4
Assisted (A)	3
Marginal (M)	2
Dependent (D)	1

Determine a cutoff value for each subscale or for the total instrument to use as a passing standard. The user might also wish to identify critical elements which must be met. Alternatively, faculty may wish to specify levels of performance (I, A, S, M, D) to be met as a passing standard for each course or level of the curriculum.
*Rating scale labels adapted from Dr. Kathleen Bondy

Clinical Competence Rating Scale

Problem Solving	I	S	A	M	D	NO NA	Comments
1. Collects relevant health data from client and other sources							
2. Assesses client's ability to communicate verbally							
3. Assesses client's physical status							
4. Assesses client's psychosocial status							
5. Assesses client's developmental level							
6. Assesses client's environmental safety needs							
7. Assess impact of illness on client and significant others							
8. Assesses learning needs of client and significant others							
9. Differentiates subjective and objective client data							
10. Interprets client's nonverbal behavior							
11. Formulates nursing diagnoses and/or problem list							
12. Seeks client input to develop a plan of care							
13. Considers client's cultural background when planning care							
14. Formulates a plan of care consistent with client's values							
15. Consults with other members of the health care team							
16. Supports client's right to a personal philosophy and lifestyle							
17. Develops rapport with client and health team members							
18. Recognizes signs and symptoms of physical distress in client							
19. Documents nursing interventions and client responses							
20. Reports pertinent client information to appropriate health team members							
21. Seeks assistance when needed							
22. Evaluates client's responses to therapeutic interventions							
23. Evaluates client's progress toward desired outcomes							
24. Revises plan of care when indicated							
25. Allows client to choose freely among alternative actions							
26. Incorporates client's significant others into plan of care when appropriate							
27. Schedules nursing activities to promote client comfort							
28. Organizes activities to promote efficiency							
29. Acts as an advocate for the client							

Clinical Competence Rating Scale

Application of Theory to Practice	I	S	A	M	D	NO NA	Comments
30. Utilizes therapeutic communication skills with client							
31. Develops a plan of care for client based on assessment data							
32. Plans nursing activities that facilitate the achievement of client outcomes							
33. Plans nursing activities that are congruent with the prescribed medical regimen							
34. Anticipates client's responses to therapeutic interventions							
35. Anticipates client's needs after discharge							
36. Implements nursing activities to meet client's needs							
37. Detects salient aspects of client's behavior							
38. Incorporates theoretical knowledge and scientific principles into nursing care							
39. Reacts to signs and symptoms of distress in client							
40. Carries out patient teaching							
41. Conveys an attitude of acceptance and empathy toward client							
42. Acts in a nonjudgmental manner toward client							
43. Maintains client/family confidentiality							
Psychomotor Skill Performance							
44. Demonstrates manual dexterity with equipment							
45. Adapts skill performance to client situation							
46. Performs skills with minimal discomfort to client							
47. Gathers necessary equipment and supplies prior to performing a skill							
48. Recognizes hazards to client							
49. Maintains client safety							
50. Maintains medical asepsis							
51. Uses sterile technique when indicated							
52. Documents nursing interventions in client record							
53. Documents client's response to nursing interventions in client record							

*Rating scale labels adapted from Dr. Kathleen Bondy

BIBLIOGRAPHY

1. Oermann MH, Gaberson KB: Evaluation and Testing in Nursing Education. New York, Springer, 1998.
2. Scheetz LJ: Development of an instrument to measure clinical competence in the baccalaureate nursing student. In Waltz C, Strickland O (eds): Measurement of Outcomes in Nursing Education and Practice, Vol. II. New York, Springer, 1990.
3. Scheetz LJ: The clinical competence rating scale—an update. In Waltz CF, Lenz ER (eds): Measurement of Outcomes in Nursing Education. New York, Springer, in press, 2000.
4. Waltz CF, Strickland OL, Lenz ER: Measurement in Nursing Research. Philadelphia, FA Davis, 1984.
5. Woolley GR, Bryan MS, Davis JW: A comprehensive approach to clinical evaluation. J Nurs Educ 37:361-366, 1998.
6. Wren KR, Wren TL: Legal implications of evaluation procedures for students in healthcare professions. AANA J 67:73-78, 1999.

17. TEACHING TO A DIVERSE STUDENT GROUP: TRANSCULTURAL CONCEPTS

Linda S. Smith, DSN, RN

1. Why should diversity concepts be used to complement and strengthen a class or clinical group?

When students perceive a difficult learning environment, it usually means the existence of conflicting cultural beliefs and values. Mere knowledge about a cultural group or race is never enough, nor does a cookbook list of cultural traits translate into actual cultural competence.

All persons have ethnicity and all persons bring to any interaction a set of beliefs and behaviors that are rooted in their family, ethnic, and cultural backgrounds. All persons (students, peers, clients) deserve to have their ethnicity valued by culturally competent educators. To ignore the different cultures and cultural needs of students would be to inadequately prepare students as team players within a multicultural society. In word and deed, educators need to recognize and appreciate the diversity in all students; the needs of each student are identified and considered individually. That means, instead of teaching about opposites, culturally competent educators teach about complements and synergy. Educators, therefore, demonstrate cultural competence as key players in the process for all interactions within nursing.

For nursing faculty, the focus is on meeting different needs of very diverse students and student groups. Indirectly, positive, honest, growth-producing relationships with diverse peers and faculty will translate into culturally competent care by all students.

2. How do I celebrate diversity versus merely managing it within our program and student groups?

First, and most important, culturally competent educators are aware of their own cultural bias, assumptions, and stereotypes; recognize these as potentially harmful to the teaching-learning process; and set them aside so as to provide the best possible learning environment for students. As population diversity continues to expand, educator commitment to diverse nursing students is the key factor to affecting a positive influence with them. This is high-level cultural awareness, otherwise known as bridging (creating culturally adaptive instructional responses-bridges-for diverse students). This means that culturally competent faculty should question everything they do in the classroom and clinical settings.

Faculty celebrate diversity by understanding that culture influences communication, perceptions of space, spatial behavior, and cultural attitudes regarding family, work, religion, and relationships. Culture greatly influences time orientation (past, present, or future). What happens when education classes must run punctually and time-efficiently? How students feel about their environments, whether they believe they are in control or are controlled by others, are important considerations for educators. Certainly, differences among races do exist; so, too, are the differences within a race or cultural group.

3. How and why do I facilitate gender and cultural conflict resolution?

Culturally competent educators attack processes, not people. They facilitate student ownership of problems and solutions, and they maintain group congruence by promoting clear objectives and goals. Importantly, educators should formally address and discuss cultural influences on conflict, reduce cultural barriers (racism, sexism, stereotyping), and plan culturally mixed activities. These activities help students feel pride in their identities and successes as well as pride in their work as group members. Faculty demonstrate problem-solving approaches by using experiences as examples, as well as by teaching and encouraging assertive behavior. Listening is the major ingredient to facilitating conflict resolution. Listen to students' experiences (be a listening role model) and work to create a respectful, listening environment for everyone.

Cultural brokerage is a nursing intervention that involves bridging, negotiating, and linking the healthcare (institutional) culture with that of the client or student. Faculties who engage in cultural brokerage will enhance cultural conflict resolution by first identifying differences between beliefs/goals of students and institutional missions, discussing, and clarifying these differences openly, and negotiating acceptable compromise.[10]

Confronting cultural insensitivity is an excellent practice. A preidentified word such as "stop" or "hurt" could be used to signal a culturally insensitive interaction. Everyone must agree that the use of this word will immediately lead to a private discussion about the incident.

4. How do I facilitate leadership among my minority students?

A mentor/mentee relationship is one excellent way to facilitate minority student leadership. Mentors/mentee dyads may attend professional meetings, ethnic nursing organizations, conferences, staff meetings, and network gatherings. Thus, mentees have opportunities to practice interpersonal skills in many settings, develop time management skills, learn current trends and issues, develop strategies for professional growth and mobility, and consider advanced nursing opportunities and education. Gender and ethnicity mentor/mentee matches are important but not essential. What is essential is an attitude of professional caring with well-planned orientation sessions for each group.

Besides developing mentoring programs, faculty should actively solicit minority students for participation in projects and organizations (at all university levels). Additionally, instructors need to respect occasions that are especially meaningful to minority students, such as the anniversary of Dr. Martin Luther King, Jr.'s birth and death, and spiritual celebrations.

5. Is it important to get our student nurse association involved?

Yes! To promote active democratic decision-making among nursing students, the program's student nurse association can and should become involved. Faculty may also facilitate the formation of minority student support groups for the purposes of peer counseling, mentoring, networking, social relations, and tutorial or study services. Loneliness leads to high rates of attrition among minority students; these informal and formal organizations facilitate resolution of personal as well as professional problems. Thus, besides creating a culturally sensitive set of bylaws and agenda, minority students will learn valuable organization and leadership skills.

6. There is so little time and so much to teach. How do I integrate diversity themes within existing program curricula?

To decrease administrative resistance and apathy, faculty will need to integrate transcultural nursing concepts within existing curricula. This can be done in the following ways:
- Using minority speakers as guest lecturers for class, institution, and organization meetings
- Describing (with demonstration) health practices of various ethnic groups during class and clinical discussions

- Creating culturally-based reading assignments that address aging and health and wellness promotion issues
- Teaching cultural diversity as part of every nursing course
  - nursing history (biographies of ethnically diverse nursing leaders worldwide)
  - health policy (access to care issues for disadvantaged groups, such as newcomers)
  - research (limited representation and ethical issues of diversity in research studies)
  - medical-surgical clinical and theory courses (cultural assessments, holistic care, culturally competent plans of care)
  - pathophysiology and physical assessment (genetic diversity)

7. What specific teaching strategies should I use with my culturally diverse students?
   Faculty teaching ethnically diverse students need to engage in the following activities on a consistent basis.
- Devote more time to explaining concepts and procedures.
- Create culturally sensitive teaching aids, such as lecture notes, handouts, audiotapes.
- Request feedback by asking, "Of the concepts we have talked about, what seems confusing, clear, difficult?" Asking "Do you understand?" is a worthless endeavor.
- During course and unit exams, allow more time per question. Also, language dictionaries are essential tools during testing sessions.
- Communicate the importance of culture to all student groups. Faculty may no longer teach to the three distinct races.
- Teach the value of journaling, family histories, and cultural autobiographies, thereby helping students recognize cultural identities.
- Teach with stories. Everyone wants to tell life stories. Support and encourage these stories during class and clinical discussions. Stories help tellers and listeners make sense of new experiences.
- Use lots of wait time (the space of time between question and answer). Increase this wait time from the usual 0.9 seconds to three or more seconds. (Refer to the chapter on Critical Thinking for further discussion on wait time.)
- Use integrated peer-teaching and student teaching. This is especially helpful for students from ethnic and gender backgrounds that value teamwork and collegial interaction.
- Listen carefully to nonverbal cues; these cues are the most important indicators of confusion. When students nod affirmatively, do not assume it means "yes." They may be nodding affirmation just to save face. Always ask open-ended questions.
- Liberally refer students to programs and college resources (colleagues, other departments, financial aid, counseling, tutoring, etc.). Follow-up on all referrals.
- Use authentic cultural artifacts as teaching/learning aids.

8. How will I know if my teaching efforts have been effective?
   Outcomes-based research is a key ingredient to measuring and tracking cultural competence strategies and diversity program success. Analyze the impact your efforts have had on:
- Recruitment and retention of ethnically diverse students
- Student satisfaction surveys during the nursing program and post-graduation
- Faculty and employer satisfaction survey
- Pre- and post-instruction or program cultural competence surveys (make sure the reliability and validity data support their use; consider Bernal and Froman's Cultural Self Efficacy Scale [CSES], 1987, 1993)

Student survey instruments need to include items assessing perceived levels of faculty and program respect, encouragement, adaptability, and support. Ask "Do ethnically diverse students believe their personal and professional needs have been met?" Additionally, programs need to survey faculty with an item such as, "To what degree are minority students viewed as positive enhancements for the class, for nursing, and for culturally competent nursing care?" Another item that can be included on a faculty survey is "To what degree are students encouraged to maintain cultural identities?"

9. Should I learn students' language?

Learning another culture is not possible until the language is also understood. Language is the transmittal tool for culture. Program staff who speak the language of students will find that rapport is enhanced. In areas of high Hispanic populations, such as Florida, Texas, and California, at least one faculty member should be fluent in Spanish. Educators in programs in or bordering Canada need French-speaking skills. Fortunately, many language courses are offered in alternative delivery format. Taking one or more of these courses will enhance cultural competence and language awareness. Language comprehension is a great gift for the instructor as well as the student.

10. How (and why) should our faculty and program improve retention of minorities?

There is a consistent pattern of high levels of attrition as culturally diverse students progress from nursing program admission to graduation. Personal issues and problems, such as loneliness and health, along with academic and time management difficulties, need to be recognized and resolved.

Barriers to minority student success are many and the first step is to identify them. How ready the student is to move into the nursing role depends on how much that student values these new behaviors and how much support is being given for these monumental changes. Additionally, barriers of time, finances, priorities, values, educational performance, and role conflict all impact student success. Though the instructor may not perceive these barriers as problems, it is the student's perception of these barriers and their consequences that make the difference.

To improve student retention, students and their families need to view all resources as culturally competent and accessible. For example, is the program perceived as supportive to minority students? Are external and internal material and financial resources available? Finally, if students decide to commit to the required behavior change, what are the benefits to them and to their families? Do these benefits outweigh the real and perceived costs?

Several retention approaches are better than a single intense focus on just one. Faculty commitment, positive, respectful teacher/student relationships, and role modeling and mentoring by minority faculty are program-wide techniques that improve minority student retention. Specific retention efforts of minority student candidates can include:

- Teaching cultural diversity as an integrated component of the nursing curriculum (the word will spread!)
- Developing flexible course scheduling, including weekends and evening classes, so that work and family roles can be maintained
- Formulating and implementing alternative delivery course mechanisms, such as Internet, audio, and video course dissemination
- Establishing on-site, inexpensive, quality-based baby sitting services
- Developing culturally competent tutoring and remediation programs
- Hiring staff from minority groups, including secretarial, counseling, administrative, and teaching staff
- Researching program problems/solutions experienced by minority students

11. How (and why) should our faculty and program increase recruitment efforts of minority candidates?

Despite the huge numbers of North American RNs, the profession is predominately Caucasian female in composition. Presently, United States registered nurse statistics demonstrate 90% white, 4% black, 3.4% Asian, and 1.4% Hispanic.[4] Clients in busy, ethnically diverse communities go to their healthcare facilities and see "white women." As with other health care professionals, registered nurses self-identifying as minority group members are more likely to practice in areas demonstrating great ethnic diversity and registered nurses shortages, especially urban, low socioeconomic communities.[5] Without ethnically diverse graduates, ethnic minorities within faculty employment pools will continue to be scarce. Without faculty mentors, role models, and counselors, ethnically diverse students will feel even more isolated. Thus, the vicious circle grows.

Recruitment efforts of minority student candidates can include:
• Developing high school tutor centers with student and faculty volunteers
• Providing these services in target community areas
• Providing ethnically diverse advisors, recruiters, and counselors for minority-based potential applicants
• Establishing programs for ethnically diverse faculty and community nursing professionals to visit and work in high schools, health and recruitment fairs, high school and college career days, and supermarket blood pressure screening booths
• Establishing scholarship programs for disadvantaged and minority students and candidates
• Writing (with careful critiques) recruitment brochures that feature minority students
• offering pre-professional courses that facilitate minority student program interest and success
• Participating with local high schools and state labor boards to establish a high school health occupations course
• Providing ethnically diverse tours, materials, learning aids, and faculty lecturers for enrollees in a health occupations course

12. Do my students experience culture shock when they enter our nursing program?

Collegiate experiences are designed to pull students away from cultural values and attitudes of families and societies. A college education is meant to broaden and liberate ideas by exposing students to new information, challenges, and perspectives. This is the culture of a nursing program. These activities, however, create dissonance between students, family, and community. Students are asked to reject and liberate their ordered thinking for the purpose of a professional career. Unfortunately, guilt and anger are almost always a side effect of this profound change due to the conflict between culture of origin and program/professional culture. This is especially true for students who self-identify with strong, distinct subculture groups. Stress, anger, and guilt will be experienced whether students reject the home culture, try to juggle (compromise) both cultures, or reject the nursing program culture. Most frequently, students choose to compromise between cultures. This is why interactions within culture groups, such as joining ethnic nursing associations, are so essential in resolving culture shock. Such associations provide a kind of rest station for students to exercise new nursing values, yet maintain their cultural identities.

13. What can I do to better prepare myself for teaching to diverse students?

Nurse educators can prepare themselves for teaching to diverse students by:
• Performing an in-depth personal cultural assessment

- Committing fully to personal and professional cultural competence
- Watching and listening to political and foreign news (preparation for analysis of global impact on health and healthcare)
- Traveling to and working in foreign countries, bringing these experiences to the classroom
- Keeping a teaching journal
- Thinking and writing about personal history and experiences
- Videotaping classes and observing for cultural insensitivities
- Learning to use technology (Internet, audiotapes, presentation software) in order to accommodate diverse learning styles
- Attending cultural competence seminars, workshops
- Reading and viewing culturally sensitive materials
- Learning new languages
- Consulting with community and professional cultural experts

14. What must I never do, whether in front of the class or at the bedside?
Faculty must *never*:
- Intimidate by appearing hurried, uncaring, closed, and frustrated
- Leave students and student groups in confused states
- Treat all students alike
- Disregard the importance of ethnicity on the teaching/learning process
- Demonstrate intolerance to cultural differences
- Expect one individual to speak on behalf of his or her entire culture
- Base all admission and progression decisions on standardized exam scores. Standardized exams most often demonstrate familiarity with middle-class Caucasian culture and do not necessarily measure actual intelligence or ability. Ask "Are these norm-referenced tests fair to minorities, women, and older students?"

15. Are there any books, videos, or Internet sites available to help me and my students more fully understand diversity issues?
Besides professional nursing and teaching resources, there are hundreds, maybe thousands, of resources that will provide faculty and students with improved levels of cultural knowledge and sensitivity. Here are a few favorites:
Internet:
   www.yforum.com (a truly excellent web site; offers an outstanding, no-holds-barred, diversity dialogue)
Print:
   The Spirit Catches You and You Fall Down (Fadiman, 1997)
   The Men with the Pink Triangle: The True Life and Death Story of Homosexuals in the Nazi Death Camps (Heger, 1994)
   I Know Why the Caged Bird Sings (Angelo, 1984)
Video:
   The Color of Fear (1994). Oakland, California: Stir-Fry Productions, by Lee Mun Wah
Popular Films:
   Hoop Dreams
   The Joy Luck Club
   Boys 'n the Hood
   The Color Purple

BIBLIOGRAPHY

1. Alvarez A, et al: Mentoring undergraduate ethnic-minority students: A strategy for retention. J Nurs Educ 32:230-232, 1993.
2. Smith LS: Trends in multiculturalism in health care. Hosp Material Management Quarterly 20:61-69, 1998.
3. Davidhizar R, et al: Managing a multicultural radiology staff. Radiology Management 19:50-55, 1997.
4. American Nurses Association [ANA] Nursing Facts: Today's registered nurse—numbers and demographics [Online]. American Nurses Association, 1994. http://www.nursingworld.org/readroom/position/index/htm.
5. Tucker-Allen S: Losses incurred through minority student nurse attrition. Nurs Health Care 10:395-397, 1989.
6. Smelser NJ: The politics of ambivalence: Diversity in the research universities [online]. American Academy of Arts and Sciences. Daedalus 122:37-53, 1993. Available: http://web.lexis-nexis.com/univers.
7. Grossman D, et al: Cultural diversity in Florida nursing programs: A survey of deans and directors. J Nurs Educ 37:22-26, 1998.
8. Razzano E: The overseas route to multicultural and international education [online]. Helen Dwight Reid Educational Foundation, The Clearing House 69:268-270, 1996. http://web.lexis-nexis.com/univers.
9. Yoder MK: Instructional responses to ethnically diverse nursing students. J Nurs Educ 35:315-321, 1996.
10. McCloskey JC, Bulechek GM: Nursing Interventions Classification (NIC): Iowa Intervention Project, 2nd ed. St. Louis, Mosby, 1996, p 193.

18. THE LEARNING RESOURCE CENTER

Kelly L. Fisher, MS, RN

1. What is the role of the learning resource center (LRC) in nursing education?

Over the years, nursing education has focused on curriculum changes that enhance critical thinking and active inquiry, rather than passive learning. From a faculty perspective, "active learning" means involvement of the students through listening and participation in activities designed to engage them in the learning process. Formerly referred to as the "skills lab," the concept has evolved to include teaching and learning in all three domains (cognitive, affective, and psychomotor). Thus, the learning resource center (LRC) is an integral part of the nursing curriculum, providing an arena for active and interactive learning, where students engage in computer work, observation, and practice of psychomotor and communication skills. The LRC is a "bridge" for students to learn and practice basic and advanced psychomotor, cognitive, and communication skills prior to entry into the clinical practice areas. The center provides a "safe" environment, with controlled variables, wherein the student can learn in a simulated practice setting. Even after students complete that first psychomotor skills course, the lab provides a safe haven for students to prepare for new experiences they will encounter in the clinical setting.

In the ideal world, students would know specifically what care will be required by their patients in the clinical setting on any given day. Prior to that day, the student would visit the LRC, complete a computer-assisted learning program, view videotapes, and practice psychomotor skills related to the care they will provide. For example, if the student will be caring for a postoperative patient with a central line and multiple medications, the student would visit the LRC the day prior to clinical, view related videotapes, complete related computer-assisted instruction, practice physical assessment and the psychomotor skills that will be used to provide care. Unfortunately, clinical practice settings are often too dynamic to enable such planned assignments by faculty and preparation by students.

To facilitate an effectively functioning LRC requires a collaborative effort between nursing course faculty and the individual responsible for operating the center. Ideally, the LRC will have its own staff, who may or may not have faculty appointments. For the efficient and effective operation of the center, someone should have full-time responsibility for the center's day-to-day operations, including purchasing, inventory, supervision of student practice, and, in some instances, testing. For the purposes of this chapter, that special "someone" who operates the center and assists students is referred to as the LRC instructor/coordinator (I/C).

2. What about the physical environment of the LRC?

The LRC should be a functional environment, providing adequate lighting, space for chairs, tables, book shelves, television, VCR, computer(s), hospital beds with privacy curtains and bedside tables, exam tables, mannequins, and anatomic models. There should be adequate space to set up equipment and supplies and to allow for necessary movement by students and faculty. Provisions should be made to secure equipment and supplies, either by storage in a locked closet or other secured area.

3. How does one set up the LRC?

Ideally, the LRC should be a large enough to accommodate 30-40 students. A multi-purpose learning resource center will have the following areas: simulated ambulatory care area, simulated hospital unit, discussion and audiovisual viewing area, computer stations, locked storage area, and sink(s) for hand washing. An area for hospital beds with privacy curtains, an overbed table, and a bedside table should be available. Actual simulation of a hospital room is very helpful, with sphygmomanometers and oxygenation/suction equipment mounted on the walls. If space allows, set up another area of the center as an ambulatory care area, complete with exam tables, scale, wall-mounted sphygmomanometers, otoscopes, and ophthalmoscopes. A separate area of the LRC should have a table and chairs so that students and the LRC I/C have a place to sit during a discussion or while viewing videotapes. Also, needed is an area with a sink for hand washing, and cabinets for the storage of small equipment and supplies. A larger locked storage closet is necessary to store expensive mannequins, bed linens, and medical equipment. If possible, develop an area for the integration of technology such as some computers for interactive learning, and a television with a VCR or other media access for viewing visual tutorials. Remember to have bookshelves in a reference area with current textbooks and course syllabi available.

4. Setting up an LRC sounds expensive! How do we find the money?

LCRs *are* expensive because of the equipment and supplies that are needed for student learning. The initial funding to set up an LRC, as described above, can be acquired through external or internal funding. Externally, private foundations might be willing to fund the establishment or refurbishing of learning resource centers whose purpose is compatible with the mission of the foundation. Internally, the college or university might be willing to appropriate strategic funds if faculty can demonstrate the relationship between the LRC and the college/university's goals and funding priorities.

Maintaining the LRC inventory, including durable equipment and disposable supplies, is costly. Mannequins and anatomical models range in price from several hundred to several thousand dollars each. Equipment such as sphygmomanometers, glucometers, ophthalmoscopes, and otoscopes must be repaired and/or calibrated from time to time. Hospital beds and other durable medical equipment can also be quite costly. Disposable patient care supplies, such as urinary catheters, dressings, intravenous fluids and tubing, needles and syringes, suction catheters, etc., can add up quite quickly. Schools have several options to defray costs: charge students a technology fee, require that students purchase a preassembled lab kit, or both. The LRC I/C is challenged to balance the need to provide students with sufficient equipment and supplies to practice as needed, while at the same time to discourage waste. Students should be aware of the cost of supplies, particularly sterile supplies, so that they will develop fiscal accountability in the lab and the practice setting.

5. What kinds of content can be taught in the LRC?

The LRC should be an integral part of all clinical nursing courses. Curriculum content that can be taught in the learning resource center includes, of course, psychomotor skills. Additional content taught in the center includes communication skills and cognitive skills, which are taught effectively through the use of role-playing and interactive technology. Basic and advanced psychomotor skills that can easily be taught in the learning center include blood pressure, patient hygiene, bed making, mobility, intravenous therapy, medication administration, oxygenation, tracheostomy care, venipuncture, specimen collection, central venous line/ PICC line care, nasogastric suction, a chest tube set up, ostomy care, bandaging, wound care, urinary catheter insertion and care, traction and cast care, medication calculations, and physical assessment (neonate, child, adult, and geriatric).

Communication skills can be taught by role playing in the center. The availability of computers, video cameras, VCRs, and other learning technology broadens the old concept of the "skills lab," so that the "lab" actually becomes an LRC. When students have access to multimedia technology in the LRC, teaching-learning occurs in all three domains.

6. What methods of instruction are appropriate for the LRC?

The methods of instruction for teaching psychomotor and communication skills include demonstrations by the LRC I/C or course faculty, return demonstrations by students, role playing, and the use of videotapes and interactive computer media. Students should be provided with adequate opportunities to practice skills with the guidance of faculty or the LRC I/C, who is available to answer questions and provide feedback to students regarding their performance. Utilizing this teaching approach fosters students' learning through active involvement with course content, equipment, and supplies.

The most effective lab instruction occurs with small groups of students. If the student group is large, several faculty should be available to teach in the learning resource center. Teaching students in groups of 6–10 persons per faculty member allows for collegiality, collaboration, close supervision, and open communication.

7. How does one set up a teaching situation in the learning resource center?

Effective implementation of student learning activities, utilizing tutorials, videotapes, interactive computer media, mannequins, anatomic models, and actual simulated performance of a skill, requires the acquisition of current equipment, supplies, and media. These things accomplished, the curriculum content to be addressed in the LRC requires specific learning objectives, method of instruction, outcomes, and an evaluation process, all of which should be shared with the LRC I/C.

Equipment and supplies should be organized for easy accessibility by faculty or the LRC I/C. It is a good idea to keep all equipment and supplies needed for a particular skill in a plastic crate or box, labeled appropriately. To set up a teaching situation, the LRC I/C or faculty should select an appropriate area for placing the mannequin or model, assemble all of the equipment necessary to review the principles and demonstrate the appropriate technique for performing the skill, and set up the videotapes or other visuals, ready to be viewed by the students. It is important when doing simulations and role playing that the equipment closely resemble the actual equipment used in clinical practice.

Begin the instruction by reviewing the principles and steps for performing the skill. Often, this is done with a brief lecture and/or a videotape. Following the skill demonstration by faculty or the LRC I/C, each student should have time to practice the skill and then return a demonstration. Return demonstrations should be supervised by the LRC I/C or faculty, and appropriate feedback given to enable students to refine psychomotor skills.

If a self-paced modular approach is used to teach psychomotor skills, students should have the objectives and assigned content for each module. The modular learning approach has specific objectives and outcomes, a list of structured activities, and a multimedia integration design. Students may move through the required clinical lab modules at their own pace.

A skills checklist can be used as a reference tool during the demonstration and as an evaluation instrument. The checklist should indicate critical elements of the skill performance. Skill evaluations, typically, are not assigned a letter grade but are graded as satisfactory or unsatisfactory. Checklists can be retained in the students permanent record by the nursing department.

8. What are the role and responsibilities of the LRC I/C?

The role of the LRC I/C may differ, depending upon whether the individual has a staff or faculty appointment. If the individual has a staff appointment, his or her role may include classroom teaching responsibilities in addition to those responsibilities involved in the day-to-day operation of the LRC. On the other hand, if the individual has a staff position, he or she may not have assigned teaching responsibilities, but will still be responsible for supervising students' practice in the LRC. Regardless of the type of appointment, the LRC I/C must work collaboratively with all nursing faculty. Since students who are enrolled in many different nursing courses will be using the LRC, the LRC I/C should have course syllabi and other pertinent references for all courses.

The LRC I/C is usually responsible for the following: scheduling appropriate time for instruction for different groups of students in various nursing courses, allotting time during the week for student practice sessions, being available during practice time and throughout the academic year to assist students, obtaining the necessary equipment and supplies and maintaining the LRC, maintaining an inventory and purchase ordering system, and developing a budget in collaboration with the nursing dean or chairperson.

Scheduling instruction time in the LRC should be done in collaboration with the faculty of each nursing course, in advance of the start of an academic year, to provide adequate time in the learning resource center for each group of students and to prevent overlaps. The LRC I/C should then designate times for practice sessions. The LRC I/C or course faculty should be available during practice sessions to assist students. The LRC should be open for student use throughout the entire academic semester so that students may return to the center during a clinical rotation if he or she desires to practice a clinical skill.

Given the nature of the LRC, the LRC I/C will be a resource person who is approachable and relates well to students. Students must feel comfortable going to the LRC for assistance with skill practice or to use other available resources. Making a connection with each student by getting to know students' names is helpful and should be done at the beginning of each academic year. Begin to assess students' learning styles, strengths, and weaknesses. Once student weaknesses are identified, the LRC I/C can work with the student to improve performance. Moreover, the LRC I/C plays a vital role in the identification of "high risk" students. In this capacity, the LRC I/C can collaborate with the student and course faculty to plan and implement activities that will improve critical thinking and psychomotor skills, thus reducing the possibility of unsuccessful program completion.

9. Should students be required to practice in the LRC outside of scheduled class time?

Yes. It is the old adage, practice makes perfect. Faculty should require students to spend time in the LRC to practice psychomotor skills and to utilize all available resources of the center. The idea of requiring the students to practice may not be their idea of fun, but often when they actually arrive at the LRC and begin to work, they begin to take their learning seriously and leave the center with increased confidence. The opportunity to practice in the LRC is advantageous for students in that it provides the opportunity to engage in peer critiquing, sharing of information, and peer support. Students engage in collaborative learning and form collegial relationships with faculty, peers, and the LRC I/C in a nonthreatening environment. The retention of information by the student is often increased with active learning in such an environment. Thus, one would expect that students' performance in clinical settings and on the NCLEX exam would be improved.

10. Should students be required to demonstrate mastery of content in the LRC prior to practicing psychomotor skills in a clinical setting?

Requiring that students be accountable for their own learning is very important in the nursing curriculum. Students are recognized as adults, responsible for learning and performing those skills necessary to practice nursing. A competent student is what all faculty strive to develop, and therefore, requiring that students demonstrate mastery of psychomotor skills is appropriate and fosters accountability. However, depending upon the complexity of the skill, there might be occasions in the clinical setting which lend themselves to teaching a new skill "on the spot." (Refer to the chapter "Clinical Teaching" for more on this topic.) Generally speaking, though, students should demonstrate mastery of psychomotor skills prior to performing them on patients. At the very least, students should have the ability to perform the skill safely, even though the student might not perform the skill with the desired level of efficiency. Regardless of how well equipped the LRC is, performing skills in a simulated setting IS NOT THE SAME as performing them on patients!

11. How can a faculty member or LRC I/C encourage students' critical thinking and problem solving abilities during LRC instruction?
One teaching approach being widely used in the classroom is the use of case studies. A "story" of an actual situation describing the clinical case, followed by application-level and analysis-level questions foster students' integration of information, problem-solving ability, and critical thinking. While used frequently in the classroom, this approach has not been widely used as a teaching strategy for the LRC. The case study approach has been useful to "attach" the nursing skill to an actual in-depth story of a real-life situation.

The connections made to theory have proved useful when the student is comprehending the patient's diagnosis and the nursing actions needed to care for the patient while performing a psychomotor skill. For example, in the case study of a patient with a pneumohemothorax, each student is asked to address a question in the case study. This strategy enables the students to assess the situation, identify the significance, and determine the appropriate nursing actions. Case studies, which can be created for each lab module, enable students to perform the related psychomotor skills and to integrate nursing theory to understand why the skill is appropriate for this patient. (Turn to Chapter 26 for a sample case study.)

12. How can I, the LRC I/C, establish rapport with students?
Develop and share the ability to laugh (at yourself, of course)! Humor can alleviate stress and anxiety in situations where the students are having difficulty performing. Allow students to share their personal insights and interpretation of the situation, and then share your lived experiences from your clinical practice. The sharing of clinical stories from an expert having had similar feelings or anxieties is a powerful tool that can be used to break down barriers to students' learning. Communication between the instructor and the student can create a safe learning environment that allows students to actively learn complex information in a very successful way.

13. Who should staff the LRC?
The personnel for the LRC varies across institutions. The LRCs are increasingly becoming a team effort, with faculty collaborating with the staff hired as the LRC I/C (or whatever other title is bestowed upon the individual). The LRC staff may have different educational backgrounds, such as baccalaureate-prepared registered nurse, librarian, master's-prepared registered nurse, teaching assistant, or systems administrator with experience working with database, web sites, or video-conferencing.

Wide variations exist in the number, titles, and salaries of the LRC staff. The position(s) are usually titled and salaried based upon educational and experiential credentials. Some academic institutions hire a full-time lab instructor, whereas others contract the position as part-time. However, a knowledgeable stable individual is required for the LRC to be successful. Because of the potential for high turnover in this position, at least one faculty or staff member should be allocated to oversee the LRC procedures.

BIBLIOGRAPHY

1. Billings DM, Halstead JA: Teaching in Nursing: A Guide for Faculty. Philadelphia, WB Saunders, 1998.
2. Bonwell CC, Eison JA: Active Learning: Creating Excitement in the Classroom (ED336049). ASHE-ERIC Higher Education Reports, Washington, DC, ERIC Clearinghouse on Higher Education, George Washington University,1991.
3. Ryan-Wenger NA, Lee EM: The clinical reasoning case study: A powerful teaching tool. Nurse Pract 22:66-85.
4. Stewart JA: Balancing learner control and realism with specific instructional goals: Case studies in fluid balance for nursing students. Medinfo, 8 Pt 2:1715, 1995.

19. INTEGRATING TECHNOLOGY IN THE CLASSROOM

Gail K. Baumlein, PhD(c), RN, CNS

1. What is technology integration?

Technology integration refers to using computers and software effectively in teaching. It is more than simply adding computer labs and buying software. It is integrating the use of computers within the curriculum to allow enhancement of student learning.

2. Why should I integrate technology into my classroom?

One of the goals of today's nurse educator is to ensure that nursing students are technologically literate. As nursing education moves into the new millennium, we need to prepare nurses who have basic computer literacy for gathering information and communicating in our electronic world. In a learning environment, computers allow real-world applications that promote critical thinking and increase academic engagement. Students are able to move beyond knowledge and comprehension to the application and analysis of information. Furthermore, students are more motivated by technology, thus increasing their academic engagement.

3. Our curriculum offers a required computer course, so why should I have to use computers in my teaching?

While a basic computer course teaches students how to use the computer, and may introduce them to several software programs, this type of course does not immerse the student in the use of technology to enhance their learning. If students do not see technology used regularly in their academic setting, they will not associate it with their learning. The student needs to view technology use as essential to the role of the nurse. Educators, as role models for future nurses, have an obligation to embrace new technology to prepare nurses for the future. For example, if we still used only glass thermometers in our nursing arts lab, what kind of example would we be setting for students who may never encounter this dinosaur in their practice? The same is true for computer technology. If we do not use it, we cannot expect our students to become proficient with it.

4. Do you have any suggestions for integrating technology into my nursing research course?

Yes. One of the most powerful uses of the computer is for gathering information, an essential part of nursing research. Teaching students how to search databases such as CINAHL or MEDLINE will enlighten them to the amount of information available. A project you could use would be to have the students "explode" or "focus" their search on a specific topic, gathering a specific number of references, and comparing the results of their search with those of their classmates.

5. How can I teach students to critically evaluate articles they gather from the Internet?

First, students need to be able to distinguish between professional databases, such as CINAHL, and the commercial web sites on the Internet. A form for evaluating web sites is a helpful tool. Students could be asked to look critically at the author, the sponsoring agency, the supporting resources, and the accuracy of information presented on a web site. The table below depicts information that students should examine when evaluating the usefulness of a web site.

Evaluating Web Sites

URL	AUTHOR	SPONSORING AGENCY	SUPPORTING RESOURCES	ACCURACY OF INFORMATION
www.nurse.com	John Jones	Best Nurse Today	XYZ Agency Nurse's Cure Student Nurse	Current; provides many links; medical support
www.fun.com	Suzy Smith	None	None	No medical support; pretty pictures

A helpful starting point is to create a list of appropriate web sites at which to initiate their search. For example, the National Student Nurses Association Web Site (http://www.nsna.org) may be helpful for students who are trying to find links to other student nurses. A notebook with copies of professional web pages can be kept in the computer lab or resource center to guide students to interesting sites.

6. What are the benefits to students if I use presentation software instead of overheads?

Colorful, attractive presentations and more stimulating environments engage students' attention and promote learning. The addition of graphic images to presentations allows students to see live pictures instead of textbook drawings. For example, when describing decubiti, a collection of photographs incorporated into the presentation is worth a thousand words. If handouts of the slide presentation are included, the students will spend less time writing down every word and more time listening and paying attention to what is being said by the speaker. Students can be encouraged to use presentation software for presenting group or individual projects, thus increasing their technical knowledge and improving their presentation skills.

7. What can I do to make my computer presentations more interesting?

Adding graphic images from the Internet is one way to include interesting and realistic pictures. Clipart illustrates text with graphic examples. Scanned photos of "real life" images, such as a client modeling an insulin pump, can be slipped into your presentation. Digitized video clips add another dimension and may be incorporated to add depth to your topic. Linking to CD-ROMs, such as BodyWorks®, allows students to see an animated human body with audio components. Students can see a heart beating and observe the flow of blood through the chambers. The addition of audio clips permits the student to hear things such as heart and lung sounds, which are almost impossible to describe simply by human voice.

8. I have an Internet connection in the classroom. How can I use this in my lectures?

Links to the Internet, imbedded in the presentation, provide access to the World Wide Web. Many personal and professional sites offer insight into the realities of dealing with health alterations. Support groups, bulletin boards, hypertext links, and research and advice sites abound. For example, if discussing cleft palate, one can link to a pediatric surgery site for actual pictures of children taken before and after cleft palate surgery. Many web sites are authored by individuals who share photographs of themselves. One such site provides over 100 pictures of a family with AIDS as they share their compelling story. These human connections are invaluable in bringing the real life aspects of a disease process to the classroom.

9. My students like to use electronic mail to communicate, but is there a way to make it more efficient?

Individual e-mail between the teacher and the student is often preferred to telephone communication; however, it may become time-consuming for the teacher if she or he has many students. A listserv is an ideal way for the teacher and students to communicate with one another. The listserv utilizes an e-mail format but is composed of only those "members" who join through the listserv manager. The teacher can pose questions to the group, requiring responses, and thus promote interaction between students. Another way of communicating through e-mail is by using an individual dialogue format, where the teacher may send the same set of questions to each student and require each student to reply to the dialogue. For example, the teacher may ask questions related to the student's progress in the course and request feedback about problems or questions. This format allows the student to post a private response to the teacher, without fear that the response will be read by the entire group, although it also means the teacher may have many responses to read.

10. What is a bulletin board and how does it work?

A bulletin board is an electronic method for posting messages. Just as you might tack a notice on the bulletin board in the hall, you might post a message to the electronic board for students to read. Students may also post information to this board. Threads or discussion topics may be posted, where each student is able to read the previous response and add his or her own response, thus continuing the discussion. Response to these discussions might be required as part of class participation.

11. What are some ideas for using my web site for the best advantage?

Your web site can be a premier way for your students to glean information about the course. The entire syllabus, including textbooks, assignment descriptions, study guides, review questions, and class outline can be included. This allows students to visit the site before the course begins to see what will be expected, and also permits prospective students to browse through the course information to help decide if this is a course they might wish to take. A well-designed web site can help to "sell" your course to prospective students. Posting examples of previous class projects or advice from previous students can provide a guide for what will be expected. The web site also provides a forum for including pertinent hypertext links to other web sites you would like students to explore. This exploration can be used as an out-of-class assignment to encourage students to expand their knowledge on the course content.

12. How can I use the computer in the classroom to help develop critical thinking skills?

The same computer-assisted instruction and software programs that students use in your computer labs can be brought into the classroom for group discussions. Many problem-based learning scenarios are available commercially, and can be projected in the classroom to practice critical thinking skills. Practice quizzes and exams are also available for classroom use. Games, such as ACLS Jeopardy®, can be downloaded or purchased and used as a base for small group or class discussion.

13. What is the best way to evaluate learning from technology?

Evaluation of learning with technology is the same as with other teaching methods. Formal course evaluations by both faculty and students, targeting the technology, will provide insight about student learning. Exam and assignment grades are also effective measurement tools. Results of standardized tests can be compared with those of students who have not used technology in the classroom. In most cases, if you ask the student to evaluate his or her learning using technology, the results will show an increase in learning.

14. Isn't it true that using technology is more time-consuming than simply preparing a lecture?

Yes, initial preparation time often increases when adding technology to your classroom presentations. The additional time involved with electronic communication is another factor noted by teachers who use e-mail. Learning new techniques can be time-consuming for the busy teacher. Some administrators allow extra time for faculty to incorporate technology in their classroom. Use of technical support personnel can help to alleviate the time problem.

BIBLIOGRAPHY

1. Cheek J, Gillham G, Mills P: Using a computerised clinical database to enhance problem-based learning strategies for second year undergraduate nursing students. Aust Electronic J Nurs Educ 2, 1999. http://www.scu.edu.au/schools/nhcp/aejne/vol2-2/v2-2jc.htm
2. Dockstader J: Teachers of the 21st century know the what, why, and how of technology integration. T.H.E. Journal Online, Jan. 1999. http://www.thejournal.com/magazine/99/jan/feat05.html
3. Frizler K: Designing successful Internet assignments. Syllabus12: 52-53, 1999.
4. Garity J: Creating a professional presentation. J Intravenous Nurs 22:81-86, 1999.
5. Klemm WR: Eight ways to get students more engaged in online conferences. T.H.E. Journal, August 1998. http://www.thejournal.com/magazine/98/aug/feature4.html
6. Rao RV, Rao LM:. Strategies that support instructional technology. Syllabus 12: 22-24, 1999.
7. Stamler L, Thomas B, McMahon S: Nursing students respond to a computer assignment. J Prof Nurs 15:52-58, 1999.
8. Wolf ZR, Donnelly G: Public speaking: content and process evaluation of nursing students' presentations. Nurse Educator 18:30-32, 1993.

20. CURRICULUM DEVELOPMENT

Beth Davies, EdD, RN

1. What is meant by curriculum?

Webster's dictionary defines a curriculum as "a set of courses constituting an area of specialization." In this book, the area of specialization is nursing, so examples and discussion will address nursing. Curriculum development can be compared to a good travel plan, with appropriate steps to be taken along the way to ensure a good vacation, or in this case, a well-developed curriculum that will meet the needs of nursing education and, most significantly, the nursing learner, whether it is in an undergraduate, graduate, staff development, or continuing education. To sum it up, curriculum can be described as planned interactions between teacher and learner.

2. How does the curriculum "fit" within the total institution and the school/program of nursing?

The curriculum encompasses several "levels" of the total educational plan of the college or university. As such, it should relate to the total institution. Begin your exploration by examining the institutional mission. (More about mission statements later.) Next, examine the mission of the nursing school or program. The nursing school/program mission should logically flow from the institutional mission, i.e., the two should be related. The philosophy of the nursing school/program is a statement of faculty's beliefs about nursing. (More about philosophy later, too.) The next step in the sequence is stating the goals of the program(s). The goals should relate to the philosophy. The curriculum flows from the goals, and, therefore, relates to the institutional mission, school/program mission, and philosophy. The actual curriculum includes the conceptual framework (more about this later, too), level objectives, course objectives, clinical objectives, and actual content that is taught. Influencing the implementation of the curriculum are the teaching methods and learning experiences. Last, but certainly not least, is evaluation, a process that measures outcomes. The figure on the next page depicts the flow of components.

3. What are the mission and its purpose?

The mission of the college or university tells us about the values and beliefs upon which the institution is based. Likewise, the mission of the nursing program tells us about the values and beliefs upon which the nursing program is based. To justify the existence of the nursing program within the college or university, there should be congruence between the nursing program's mission and that of the parent institution. The mission of the nursing program is the charge from which your curriculum is developed.

4. What is included in a philosophy?

The philosophy of the nursing program reflects the faculty's beliefs and reasoning about the discipline of nursing, its relationship to health, society, and humankind, as well as the process of teaching and learning. Frequently, we find nursing program philosophies addressing the concepts of person, environment, health, nursing, teaching, and learning.

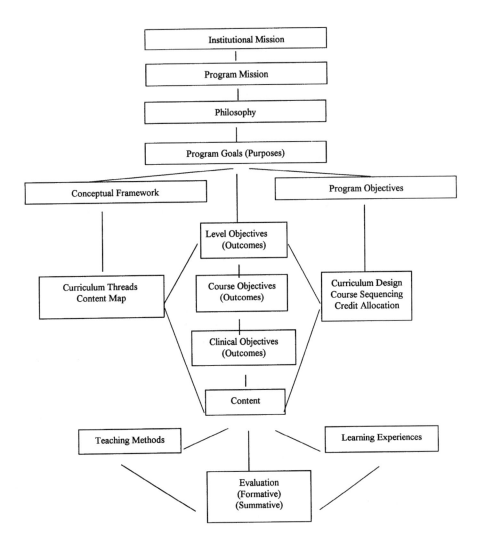

5. So where do I begin with curriculum development?

Curriculum development is an orderly process, derived, as noted in question 2, from the mission of the institution and the school/program of nursing. Therefore, to begin developing the curriculum, an examination of the institutional and nursing program missions, nursing program philosophy, and goals is the necessary first step. Next, determine a conceptual basis for the curriculum.

To use the vacation analogy, when making travel plans, you look for a place that reflects your interests and values; gather all the information you can find to inform your expectations, identify what is important to visit, and obtain maps for where you will travel. You read authoritative reports about the area and talk to friends who know the area or have been there. In the same manner, when developing curriculum, you gather all the information and develop a plan that will guide the teacher in meeting the students' needs.

6. Who develops the curriculum of a nursing program?

Faculty develop the curriculum of the nursing program. Guided by authoritative sources and professional guidelines (remember the travel guides and road maps), the faculty decide what and how the curriculum will be developed.

7. What are some of the important guidelines to be considered when developing the curriculum?

Helpful guidelines include the following publications:

- *Criteria and guidelines for the evaluation of baccalaureate and higher degree programs* (NLN)
- *Curriculum building in nursing* (NLN)
- *A vision for nursing education* (NLN)
- *Standards of practice* (ANA)
- *Roles and responsibilities for nursing continuing education and staff development across all settings* (ANA)
- *Cultural diversity in the nursing curriculum* (ANA)
- *The essentials of baccalaureate education* (AACN)
- *The essentials of master's education for advanced practice nursing* (AACN)
- *Standards for accreditation of baccalaureate and graduate nursing education* (AACN)
- *Educational mobility, vision of baccalaureate and graduate nursing education: The next decade* (AACN position paper)
- *Nursing education's agenda for the 21st century* (AACN position paper)

Also, don't forget your state's Nurse Practice Act and state Department of Education's requirements. Using professional resources establishes the credibility of your curriculum.

8. What is meant by the "core curriculum"?

The core curriculum refers to courses that contain content that is considered essential to all students that often lay ground work for courses to come in various majors. For example, English courses may be required for all students. If the college has a statement about Judeo-Christian values in its mission statement, there will probably be at least one or two religion or philosophy courses in the core. Core courses are also known as general education requirements and foundation requirements.

9. What is the purpose of the conceptual framework?

Remember your vacation planning? Part of the planning was deciding where you wanted to go and why, how you would travel, and the itinerary you would follow. Are you taking a trip that will focus on photography? If so, you will plan key places to visit, and the amount of time there will depend on how much you want to see in that area. In the same manner, when planning your curriculum, you will develop a framework with key concepts in mind, guiding the construction of courses and content. A conceptual framework serves as the basis for your curriculum planning.

10. Is there only one way to construct the curriculum?

No. Curriculum evolves through the processes that we have discussed, but the conceptual framework will determine how the actual courses will develop. With the expanded development of nursing theory, and the ever-expanding knowledge base, you can develop courses that are integrated in many ways. Depending on the nursing theorist you may want to use and the key concepts you plan to integrate, your course content may be presented in a variety of ways. Remember that this is a faculty plan with input from all nursing faculty members. Individual course development may be done by faculty with expertise in that area, incorporating threads and themes agreed upon by all the faculty.

11. What is the purpose of "leveling" objectives?

As you develop your curriculum, the complexity of the information and the skill level of your students will increase. By identifying clearly the behavioral objectives for each level, you can readily identify the progression of your student through formative and summative evaluation.

12. In the curriculum, what is the difference between course and clinical objectives?

The course objectives refer to the clearly identified behavioral statements about what the student should be able to do at the completion of the course. These include didactic information gained as well as performance expectations. Clinical objectives are clear, leveled behaviors that the student should be able to perform or exhibit in the clinical area at the completion of the course. It is important that the objective, or outcome, as it is more recently being referred to, is behavior oriented and refers to the learner.

13. What are content maps and how do they help in developing the curriculum?

Content maps help the faculty view the overall content of the curriculum and place all the content in the courses at an appropriate level. For example, faculty identify where course content is introduced and assure that those curriculum threads or themes are addressed in each course and that necessary information is "mapped" into the appropriate course. In developing the overall content map, do not go into great detail, but identify major themes and content. For example, a content map identifies where students will learn about health promotion and illness prevention, illness, childbearing, and other important content.

14. What are the differences between objectives and outcomes?

In the more recent literature, "outcomes" are being used more frequently than behavioral "objectives." The term outcomes implies that the result is more clearly defined and measurable, and places a greater learner orientation on the results. The word outcome has come into education from the business world, where quality assurance and quality improvement have become passwords of the whole health care field. Therefore, you will see course outcomes used in place of behavior objectives, since they can be more specific, with critical elements that clearly identify what is to be measured and evaluated.

15. How do threads and themes fit into the curriculum?

Your curriculum needs to fit together to create a clear picture of program content. This is accomplished by your conceptual framework. A descriptive way of weaving the tapestry together is by means of threads or themes. Though the terms horizontal and vertical threads are not used as much in recent curriculum literature, this author finds them helpful in describing how they are used. Horizontal threads are themes that are repeated across courses, with application related to content in the course. For example, if death and grieving are a horizontal thread, they may be addressed relative to the elderly in a geriatric course, while death and grieving in the loss of a child may be covered in a pediatric course. Vertical threads build on previous learning, with increased information and skill expectation expected at higher levels. For example, one of the beginning nursing courses may be physical assessment, where the basic skills are learned, whereas courses at a higher level may focus on increased skill and interpretation. Themes carry the same concept as threads, with leveling of courses and content maps determining the continuity and level of the themes.

16. What should a baccalaureate curriculum accomplish?

A baccalaureate curriculum should prepare a nurse generalist with a foundation in the liberal arts, providing the ability to apply critical thinking and problem solving to his or her practice. Furthermore, the curriculum should prepare a beginning practitioner with leadership skills and a commitment to lifelong learning. The curriculum should also develop beginning skills in research and the ability to apply theory to practice. The baccalaureate curriculum must be flexible enough to allow for change and to involve the student in his or her own learning.

17. How does the curriculum of an associate degree program differ from that of a baccalaureate program?

Length is an obvious answer, but to determine the content differences, we need to examine the program objectives. In theory, associate degree nurses are prepared to function at a technical level of practice, whereas the baccalaureate nurse is prepared for a professional level of practice. An examination of Mildred Montag's original concept of the associate degree nurse (a concept that was developed to address a nursing shortage by preparing a technical nurse in a shorter period of time, still in a collegiate setting) reveals that this nurse was educated to perform technical bedside nursing under the direction of a baccalaureate or higher level nurse. Generally speaking, Montag envisioned the associate degree nurse as one who had a more limited breadth and depth of knowledge and could provide care for patients with easily defined, predictable trajectories of illness. In contrast, the baccalaureate-prepared nurse is educated to provide care to patients with more complex, unpredictable illness trajectories. Moreover, there is additional emphasis in baccalaureate curricula on health promotion, risk identification, and illness prevention. However, the service sector rarely differentiates nursing practice in this way, so that, in many health care settings, a nurse is a nurse is a nurse. Montag's concept of the associate nurse functioning under the direction of a professional nurse is modeled on similar practices in other health professions, such as physical therapy.

While the associate degree nurse has a more limited basic education, many opportunities exist for career mobility through the development of articulation agreements with baccalaureate and graduate nursing programs. This is accomplished through the use of proficiency or placement testing in nursing knowledge and skill, and the addition of transition courses. Additional courses that may be included at the upper division level include nursing theory, research and research design, professional issues, and community health.

18. What are recent trends in curriculum development?

Curriculum development is a dynamic process. The amount of knowledge we have available increases exponentially, with information quickly becoming obsolete. Decisions must be made regarding which content to include and which to eliminate. Moreover, the focus of nursing education has shifted from process-oriented to competency-oriented, thus the emphasis on outcomes.

Recent trends promulgated by the American Association of Colleges of Nursing for baccalaureate education include an increased focus on values and ethics, reaffirmation of the importance of a liberal arts foundation in providing care that is globally relevant, increased emphasis on technology and information management, increased emphasis on leadership and management of patient care, and increased emphasis on the economics and business of health care. Cultural issues, case management, environmental issues, international health, and alternative medicine are all finding their way into curricula. Generally speaking, curriculum development is becoming increasingly integrated, with the focus more on concepts rather than on the clinical site or medical model.

Recent trends in associate degree education include an increased emphasis on care in the home and community settings, and on leadership concepts.

Trends in teaching methods include the introduction of problem- or case-focused learning. With this method, classes are not structured in the traditional lecture format. A student or group of students are given a case scenario and have to sort through information, research all the questions that arise, research the case, and develop a plan. The faculty member facilitates learning by being available for suggestions and direction, but the students are responsible for their own learning. Assigning a case study to a student team fosters the development of group cooperation and collaboration, and communication and leadership skills.

Students are increasingly involved in curriculum development and revision and policy formation. As such, curriculum needs to be fluid and flexible to meet students' learning needs. The curriculum should offer students options to meet the course objectives. In keeping with current health trends, clinical experiences will be more community oriented, and sites for clinical experiences will be more varied from the conventional hospital experiences.

As you have learned, curriculum development is evolutionary, with the need for ongoing evaluation to ensure relevance in a rapidly changing health care environment.

19. What is meant by "evidence-based practice"?

Chances are, you are familiar with this term as it relates to nursing practice. Relative to nursing education, evidence-based practice is another way of looking at nursing education and its relationship to practice. It addresses essential questions such as: What is an essential outcome of the course? Where will it be measured—in class or clinical? It includes theory, research, experience, and student self-reflection with both clinician and *patient* input. It enables the student to focus on self-evaluation of care and ongoing improvement.

20. Where does curriculum evaluation fit in?

All along the way! Faculty should continuously evaluate the curriculum. Changes should not be made without sound consideration and planning. The goal of ongoing evaluation is to maintain relevancy and current practices; evaluation is necessary to confirm your curriculum and to identify areas for improvement. Ongoing feedback allows for consistent improvement and for a realistic evaluation of how the program is meeting its stated goals and objectives.

21. Can faculty establish a totally new curriculum?

Yes. As long as the faculty can demonstrate that their approach and thinking are congruent with state education, board of nursing, and program accreditation requirements, and as long as they demonstrate sound evaluation of their program objectives, faculty can determine their own curriculum. Remember, professional organizations such as the American Nurses Association, the American Association of Colleges of Nursing, and the National League for Nursing are *not prescriptive* but, rather, provide guidelines for curriculum development. The rest is up to you!

BIBLIOGRAPHY

1. Accreditation Committee, Council of Baccalaureate and Higher Degree Programs: Criteria and Guidelines for the Evaluation of Baccalaureate and Higher Degree Programs in Nursing. New York, National League for Nursing Press. Pub. No. 15-2474, 1996.
2. American Association of Colleges of Nursing: Nursing Education's Agenda for the 21st Century. Washington, DC, 1993. http://www.aacn.nche.edu/Publications/positions/nrsgedag.htm
3. American Nurses Association: Roles and Responsibilities for Nursing Continuing Education and Staff Development Across All Settings. Washington, DC, 1992
4. American Nurses Association: Cultural Diversity in the Nursing Curriculum. Washington, DC, 1986
5. American Association of Colleges of Nursing: Essentials of Baccalaureate Education for Nursing. Washington, DC, 1998.
6. Montag M: The Education of Nursing Technicians: New York, John Wiley & Sons, 1951.
7. National League for Nursing: A Vision for Nursing Education. New York, 1993.
8. National League for Nursing: Trends in Contemporary Nursing Education. New York, Pub. No. 14-2581, 1995.

21. TEACHING AND EVALUATING CRITICAL THINKING

Ann M. Gothler, PhD, RN

TEACHING CRITICAL THINKING

1. Why is it important to define critical thinking?

Critical thinking is the foundation of professional nursing practice and an expected outcome of nursing education. As such, faculty teach critical thinking throughout the curriculum and measure it, or attempt to measure it, to document program effectiveness. Therefore, defining critical thinking becomes both a teaching and a measurement issue. Without defining what critical thinking is, there would be little congruence in the way in which critical thinking is taught. Moreover, without a clear definition of the concept, one cannot hope to measure it in any way that is meaningful.

2. So then, what is the best definition of critical thinking?

There is no "best" definition of critical thinking because the process depends on the context in which it is to be utilized. However, it is important to develop or adopt a definition of critical thinking that recognizes an ongoing lifetime process, that fits the appropriate context of nursing, and that is appropriate for the level of the learner. The literature presents varied definitions of critical thinking, most of which emphasize the reflective nature of the process, and using systematic, analytical approaches. Paul offers the following definition of critical thinking:

> Critical thinking is the intellectually disciplined process of actively and skillfully conceptualizing, applying, analyzing, synthesizing, or evaluating information gathered from, or generated by, observation, experience, reflection, reasoning, or communication, as a guide to belief and action.[4]

This definition focuses on a hierarchy of intellectual processes, similar to Bloom's taxonomy of the cognitive domain, and adds the process of obtaining the information. Paul's definition also recognizes that this process becomes the basis for decision making and the development of attitudes or beliefs. Therefore, it is especially relevant for nursing education.

3. We have been using the nursing process, nursing care plans, and clinical pathways when we teach. Doesn't that bring critical thinking into the learning process?

Not usually. In curriculum literature, critical thinking is most often used as an example of the "null curriculum"—the curriculum that we all think we are doing, but in fact are not doing. Critical thinking needs to be *explicitly discussed* and *reflected upon* by the learner in order for it to occur.

The traditional nursing process and nursing care plans are so structured and carefully described in the textbooks that they rarely allow for critical thinking without extensive faculty adaptation in their teaching approach. Nursing process and nursing care planning are very linear in their approach. Furthermore, there are many available standard care plans (or clinical pathways) which facilitate a "cookbook" approach. Clinical pathways, which have replaced nursing care plans in many hospitals, encourage even more of a "cookbook" approach than do standard nursing care plans. When there is an available answer or solution to a problem, critical thinking is often not done.

4. Why is a linear thinking approach criticized as a way to develop critical thinking skills?

Educators have long criticized the linear decision making approach of the nursing process because patient care decisions do not follow a linear trajectory. In fact, variables arise all the time that require the nurse to intervene and make other decisions prior to completing an extensive assessment of the patient. Professional nursing practice elicits ongoing feedback from each patient interaction, interactions with significant others, and from forces within the health care system. Therefore, while nurses use the skills of assessment, analysis, planning, intervention, and evaluation, these skills are often not used as a linear approach since the practice setting requires flexibility and adaptation.

It is imperative that students learn to think more like experts in order not to get bogged down doing a complete assessment, analysis, and planning prior to intervening with each patient. This does not mean that students should never do a complete assessment and planning prior to caring for the patient. Students do need to learn this process, and they also need to learn the value of decision making with an adequate database. However, equally important, students must be cognizant that they will not be able to follow a linear thinking approach with every patient because of time constraints, urgency of the patient's condition, and other variables in the practice setting. This is where critical thinking is vitally important—learning activities need to focus on selecting what do *in client-specific situations* and helping students to carefully and critically analyze alternative strategies.

5. In general, what teaching approach is needed to facilitate critical thinking?

Thinking actively and *thinking for ourselves* is most important! This concept of active thinking-active learning is very important in teaching and has been documented as more effective for all learning. In planning learning activities, keep in mind that students need to be involved in doing something *with* the ideas and concepts you want them to learn. Efforts should be directed toward having each student think through the implications, applications, utilization, and quality of the ideas that are considered. Students need to evaluate the quality of the decisions and ideas presented by faculty, peers, and others.

The following scenario is one example of a strategy used to teach critical thinking. Your students have just completed a unit on renal disease and are moving on to learn about the care of a patient with burns. When you assign the reading, you focus students' thinking with a written assignment. Some questions that you use to focus students' critical thinking include:

- How is the care of the client with third-degree burns similar to care of the patient with renal failure?
- Contrast the differences in the care of the patient with renal disease and that of a patient with burns.
- What are the major concerns of the patient and family in the acute phase (or rehabilitation phase) of the clinical problem?

Students are instructed to answer these questions through their reading, and to think about and analyze the reading material. (To facilitate critical thinking, you have ascertained that the questions are not specifically answered in the assigned reading.) You assign students to small groups so that they can get together, analyze each of their major ideas, and present their summary to the rest of the class. To further develop critical thinking skills, you vary this approach each week, using slightly different questions.

6. What are the characteristics of a learning situation which requires critical thinking?

- Exploring the situation or issue carefully

- Discussing ideas in an organized way
- Supporting ideas with evidence and reasons
- Demonstrating openness to new ideas and different viewpoints
- Challenging assumptions that form the basis for ideas, plans, clinical approaches, etc.
- Imagining and exploring alternatives—it is very important not to grab the first solution, which is often done by nurses and nursing faculty. "No-brainer" solutions usually are those in which no thought is involved, and there usually is a better solution available when the brain is involved!
- Utilizing logical reasoning skills
- Reflective learning
- Asking and answering the question, "What is the purpose of my thinking?", using an analytical approach

7. How can I improve my lectures to ensure that students learn critical thinking?

You probably can't, since critical thinking is not learned by lecture. The most faculty can do in a lecture is talk about what critical thinking should look like and focus on the need for analytical thinking in all aspects of nursing. A good lecture might sometimes reflect the faculty's development of critical thinking, but not the student's. Research has shown that listeners, on average, have about 10 minutes of attention time for content delivered by a lecture. After that, their minds wander to other thoughts (such as planning for their evening and other activities) intermittently, or for longer periods.

In order to facilitate critical thinking in your course, decrease lecture time to about 20% of the class time. Use the additional time for student participation in critical thinking activities. Courses and clinical seminars or conferences that focus on the process of caring for patients should be particularly concerned with minimizing lecture and increasing students' active learning and analytical approaches. Students need to progress through increasingly difficult critical thinking experiences.

8. What approaches can be used to develop students' critical thinking skills?

- "Advance organizers" are an important part of the introduction of a class, clinical conference, or seminar. These organizers provide connections for students from a familiar prior experience to the thinking needed in the current learning situation. The more connections or links the student has, the more retention the student will have. Sometimes faculty need to point out these connections for students, e.g., "Now that you have completed anatomy and physiology, this physical assessment course will focus on the detection of normal and abnormal functioning of the body."
- Case sets. Cognitive psychology has shown us that in our long-term memory, we remember information in narrative format (paragraphs, not lists of information). The use of case sets of examples (such as patient situations or nurse decisions) is particularly helpful for remembering clinical situations. Students, faculty, and nurses need to be encouraged to share case sets in class, clinical conferences, or informal discussion. The clinical post-conference is a very valuable time to do this, since students and faculty are rich with case examples at that moment.
- Post-conferences can focus on a topic such as the teaching-coaching role of the nurse, intervening with clients with immobility or wound management. However, this is not a good time to present new content. If students know the focus of the conference, they can then share case examples related to the topic. However, if unique case examples have occurred that day during the clinical experience, these should be valued, shared, and analyzed by all students as a first priority.

9. Shouldn't I be asking a lot of questions in class and clinical?

Yes, you're right! The use of questions as a teaching method is known as the Socratic approach. Faculty and student questions are an important part of developing critical thinking. However, the questions need to be different from the typical questions that are asked in interactions with students. If you have a specific answer in mind, you are not asking a question that will generate critical thinking. Critical thinking questions should not ask for rote recall answers or specific information. Critical thinking questions need to be broad, open questions for which the answers could go in a number of directions; these questions require analysis, new ideas, and solutions.

When you ask a question, check your watch to be sure you wait about 30 seconds before you break the silence with another question or further information. (Thirty seconds can feel like an hour when you are teaching!) Research has shown that faculty typically wait less than 5 seconds before interrupting students' thoughts on a question. This short "wait time" communicates that you do not expect deep thinking or analysis of the question.

Try keeping a set of 3" x 5" file cards, with a student's name on each card. When you ask a question, shuffle the cards, select one, and ask the student whose name is on the card to respond. Students then expect to participate at any time and tend to listen more carefully. If a student does not wish to respond, you can let him or her "pass" with the understanding that consistent nonparticipation may (or will) affect the grade.

10. How can we teach critical thinking in staff development and continuing education?

Because critical thinking is a lifelong process, we need to rethink our approach to teaching in continuing education and staff development. Often, we have focused on information transfer in a lecture lasting hours, or even all day long, to tired nurses! Yet 50% of the information learned in this format will be forgotten in a week, and 90% will be forgotten in a year unless there is adequate reinforcement. Moreover, the "necessary" information to be taught doubles every 9 months, and much nursing information is obsolete in 18 months.

Using a critical thinking approach, such as case studies or open-ended questioning, provides the opportunity for nurses to become actively involved in thinking analytically about nursing practice, including new equipment orientation and the mandated continuing education areas, such as infection control. This process helps to increase effectiveness in clinical problem solving and adapting to the changing demands of nursing practice.

EVALUATING CRITICAL THINKING

11. How can I tell when I am successful in developing students' critical thinking skills?

Analyze the students' processes of learning in your classes and clinical areas. What are they doing and thinking in the classroom? This type of thinking develops best in an atmosphere of dialogue, interchange, and problem solving. Are you and your students asking "why" and "why not" questions?

The development of critical thinking is a lifelong process for each of us. As we continue to develop new areas of expertise and adapt to the rapidly changing environment of practice, we all need these thinking skills to analyze and evaluate the vast array of health care information.

12. How can I evaluate whether someone is engaged in critical thinking?

Evaluating critical thinking requires an approach that differs from traditional testing. Much of our traditional testing focuses on recall and recognition of material that is "covered" in class, in reading assignments, and from other learning activities.

In order to evaluate critical thinking, learners need to demonstrate their ability to analyze and/or use the information in a new context. The answers cannot be found directly in class notes, or a textbook, readings, or any other learning resources. Therefore, asking open-ended questions for which several (or many) answers are possible is a good strategy to evaluate critical thinking. When evaluating the students' responses to questions, look for a logical thought process, rationale for one's decisions, and creativity.

13. How will students react to this approach to evaluation?

This evaluation approach should not be a surprise. It should reflect critical thinking that has been actively and consciously taking place in the classroom and clinical setting. Remember, in class and clinical, faculty are encouraged to ask open-ended questions and use case sets to foster critical thinking. So, when you give tests that include open-ended questions and case sets, students will be accustomed to this approach!

It is important to use a considerable amount of class and clinical conference time to help students develop the ability to analyze situations and propose creative solutions. Divergent thinking, analytical thinking, and reflective analysis are ways that students learn to think critically and creatively, and therefore should be built into the evaluation plan.

Critical thinking should be identified in writing as an important course outcome and should be reflected in written outcomes/objectives of all courses. The evaluation of critical thinking, then, reflects the expectations of the course as well as the practice environment.

14. Is it possible to use multiple-choice questions to measure critical thinking?

Yes, it definitely is possible to use multiple-choice questions to measure critical thinking. However, these questions are difficult to develop in a way that really requires students to use critical thinking skills. Moreover, "teaching to the test," as some faculty are inclined to do, changes what would have been critical thinking questions, to questions that measure only recall.

About 90% of typical multiple-choice questions are recall-recognition items which, by definition, do not measure critical thinking ability. Recall/recognition types of questions tend to be very content-focused and dependent on rote memory rather than focused on analysis and synthesis abilities.

A unique attribute of multiple-choice questions is that, by design, the question format forces the students to select one of a given series of answers. This alone stifles creativity and critical thinking. Students who have highly developed critical thinking skills might very well think of better answers that are not listed as distractors.

15. How can you tell if a test item measures critical thinking?

Often, you cannot tell just by looking at the test question, even if the question is written at the analysis level. Questions written at the recall and comprehension levels are not critical thinking questions. You need to know the context of the question within the classroom and clinical learning activities, assignments, and course-related discussion. If the content has been specifically covered in any of the learning activities, then even the "highest level" critical thinking question becomes a recall-recognition question. Any time the student has similar experiences or the material is "covered" in class or in other areas of the course, the test item then measures a lower level of cognitive learning, such as recall, recognition, comprehension, or application. If the student has been "given" the answer or has seen similar answers, the student's thinking converts to rote memory.

Critical thinking items need new solutions that require analysis in order to move beyond what is known to the unknown (answer). As you read an item ask yourself, "What type of thinking will students need to use to arrive at an answer?" If your only answer to the question is, "They need to remember that . . . ," you might have a recall-type item.

16. How do I develop test questions that measure critical thinking?

One way to develop a critical thinking question is to present a patient situation that combines a few unique clinical problems so that students are required to analyze what they have learned. The answer could focus on the best combination of clinical approaches or analysis of what information would be needed to make a decision. This type of question takes a while to develop and refine so that it measures what you intend to measure. However, once written and refined, these questions are easy to grade and provide a great assessment of the student's critical thinking skills.

Essay questions are growing in popularity in an effort to measure critical thinking. This type of question provides the opportunity for reflective thinking, creative solutions, combining ideas, analysis of assumptions, and many other skills that are part of critical thinking. Essay questions are easier to write than are multiple-choice questions; however, they take longer to grade and present more of a challenge to grade consistently.

17. Should I evaluate critical thinking in the clinical area?

Most definitely! The clinical practice environment is where the development of critical thinking should be emphasized as it relates to clinical decision making and the development of clinical judgment. Assignments that develop the quality of and extend the range of critical thinking skills enhance students' abilities to develop keen clinical judgment. Likewise, clinical evaluation methods that provide feedback about students' critical thinking enhance the development of these skills.

Faculty need a clear understanding of how each learner makes clinical decisions. Written assignments and journals that focus on students' intuitive and reflective thinking can be used to evaluate critical thinking and clinical decision making. These assignments should be evaluated on the basis of the effective use of reflective analysis (to summarize clinical experiences). Faculty can evaluate reflective analysis in students' journals and in clinical conferences.

18. Isn't it difficult to evaluate students' critical thinking in the clinical area?

Yes, because typical clinical evaluation instruments do not focus on the quality of thinking. Beyer[3] suggested that faculty consider the following questions when evaluating students' critical thinking skills. These questions could be adapted for clinical evaluation by rewording the questions into performance statements.

- How does the student develop answers to problems?
- What does the student do when he or she doesn't know the answer?
- Does the student cite reasons and sources?
- Does the student ask for reasons? Ask why?
- Does the student seek information in making decisions?
- Does the student generate many alternatives before choosing a solution?
- Does the student recognize discrepancies in the environment?

Rating students' performance on each statement, using a 5-point scale that compares students with the expected level of performance for the particular course, could be the basis of evaluating students' abilities to think creatively in the clinical setting. One example of a 5-point scale is:

1 = unsatisfactory
2 = adequate
3 = satisfactory
4 = good
5 = excellent

19. How can I evaluate critical thinking in written assignments?

Numerous criteria for evaluating critical thinking in a written assignment have been identified by Paul[4]. These questions include:

- Is the paper consistent with its stated purpose?
- Does the paper identify irrelevant concepts and ideas?
- Does the paper clarify implications of reasoning?
- Does the paper make clear and consistent inferences related to the stated purpose?
- Does the paper demonstrate evidence of logical reasoning?
- Does the paper demonstrate awareness of key concepts and ideas?
- Are there clear, consistent inferences?
- Does the paper present conclusions that are reasonable, given the information in the
  paper?

A holistic, qualitative approach is useful for grading critical thinking. For example, a
qualitative approach to grading a term paper would examine how well the total paper
expresses the author's thesis, and so on. In contrast, a quantitative approach generally
divides the paper into sections, assigning a specified number of points to each section. What
often happens when using a quantitative approach is that points are awarded for the presence of information rather than for the quality of how that information relates to the overall
thesis of the paper. In this way, the practice of grading written assignments using a quantitative approach can obstruct the evaluation of the quality and connectedness of thinking.
Students often write very good individual sections, but the quality of thinking and analysis
may not be high in the paper as a whole. If the identified ideas presented in the paper are
not significant and/or the subsequent parts do not relate to the overall purpose of the paper,
then paper should not be evaluated as one of quality.

20. How can critical thinking be rewarded?

Because the development of critical thinking skills is a valued activity, it should be rewarded appropriately. Since you have identified the value of critical thinking in your syllabus and
class discussions, and developed course outcomes and assignments that reflect critical thinking,
the next step is to assign numerical value to critical thinking assignments. Grades for critical
thinking activities should be weighted significantly to arrive at the course grade.

21. Critical thinking is so complex. How can I possibly evaluate students' thinking and acquire information that is needed for program evaluation?

The most effective evaluation approach is one of triangulation, a multifaceted approach.
This approach uses a variety of strategies that "look at" the target from differing viewpoints.
This total picture is more holistic and is usually the best estimate of the "true" characteris-
tic that you wish to measure.

In developing an evaluation plan using triangulation, you will need to select a variety
of instruments or methods to gather information about individual learners. Methods that
focus on the quality of critical thinking are presented in the table on the next page.

The evaluation plan should consist of a selected group of data collection methods from
which information can then be extrapolated to provide evidence of individual and aggregate
development of critical thinking skills. These data can be compared by individual learner
characteristics, different curricular pathways, and any other intervening variables that seem
important for your program evaluation and decision making.

22. There are so many ways to evaluate critical thinking. How do you make decisions about what approach to use?

The evaluation approach needs to match your program's needs, resources, and goals. A

word of caution—do not over-evaluate! Often there is so much material collected for evaluation that it is difficult to analyze and even more difficult to integrate the findings into curricular decision making. It is important to collect meaningful data that can be used for individual student evaluation and curricular decision making.

Methods of Evaluating Critical Thinking

EVALUATION METHOD	PURPOSE
Observation instruments	Group discussion, classroom presentations, clinical laboratory
Survey instruments (questionnaires)	Ask students, alumni, faculty, employers about critical thinking abilities of students/alumni
Structured or unstructured interviews	Ask students, alumni, and employers to evaluate critical thinking of students/alumni
Standardized examinations	Administered at program entrance and graduation to measure critical thinking ability
Journals and narratives	Provide a reflective summary of students' critical thinking; may include an exemplar
Simulations	Establish a realistic context in which to evaluate critical thinking in a controlled situation
Short analytical assignments, written summaries	Require students to summarize and prioritize information in one page
Portfolios	Provide examples of critical thinking that reflect the student's progress in the program.

BIBLIOGRAPHY

1. Alfaro-Lefevre R: Critical Thinking in Nursing: A Practical Approach, 2nd ed. Philadelphia, WB Saunders, 1999.
2. Aquilino ML: Cognitive development, clinical knowledge, and clinical experience related to diagnostic ability. Nurs Diag 8:110-119, 1997.
3. Baker CR: Reflective learning: A teaching strategy for critical thinking. J Nurs Educ 35:1 19-22, 1996.
4. Barnes CA (ed): Critical Thinking: Educational Imperative. New Directions for Community Colleges, 77, Spring, San Francisco, Jossey Bass, 1992.
5. Beyer BK: Practical Strategies for the Teaching of Thinking. Boston, Allyn and Bacon, 1987.
6. Boostrom R: Developing Creative and Critical Thinking: an Integrated Approach. Lincolnwood, IL, National Textbook Company, 1994.
7. Brookfield S: On impostership, cultural suicide, and other dangers: How nurses learn critical thinking. J Cont Educ Nurs 24:197-205, 1993.
8. Case B: Walking around the elephant: A critical thinking strategy for decision making. J Cont Educ Nurs 25: 202-210, 1994.
9. Critical Thinking Community, Sonoma State University, Rohnert Park, CA. Available: www.critical-thinking.org
10. Paul RW: Critical Thinking: How to Prepare Students for a Rapidly Changing World. Santa Rosa, CA, Center for Critical Thinking, 1993.

22. DEVELOPING WRITTEN ASSIGNMENTS

Ann M. Gothler, PhD, RN

1. Why is it important to make written assignments in my course?

Assignments focus your students on the important ideas of the course. In so doing, they are an effective method for reinforcing the assimilation of major concepts. Carefully thinking about and analyzing what is to be learned facilitates long-term memory of the material. Written assignments enable students to integrate material which they have read and discussed in preparation for application in the clinical setting. Well-constructed written assignments facilitate development of the cognitive skills of application, analysis, synthesis, and evaluation—skills that are important for critical thinking in the practice setting.

2. What are the reasons for making written assignments?

The major reasons for making written assignments include:
- To prepare for each class or clinical lab
- To enable students to focus their reading, thinking, and analysis on the important ideas in order to facilitate learning beyond the knowledge level
- To evaluate students in a specific class, the course, or clinical learning activity

3. What is my responsibility when making assignments in my courses?

Judiciously selecting assignments for your courses is a critical part of your faculty responsibility. Since the amount of content to be learned in each subject area is rapidly increasing, the selection of assignments has become extremely important and offers the hope that students will develop the ability to think and learn like a nurse. Therefore, the careful selection of the type and quantity of assignments should focus students on thinking about and analyzing the important content of the desired learning areas. When students are assigned large volumes of reading without a complementary written assignment to focus the thinking, they often experience difficulty determining what is most important and least important within the assigned reading. So then, your responsibility as a teacher is to develop assignments that focus students' thinking on key concepts of the course.

4. How do I determine the "right" number of assignments for my course(s)?

The expectation is that faculty will make assignments in relation to the number of hours or credits per course. Assignments include reading textbooks and related literature, viewing videotapes, completing computer-assisted instruction, self-practice in the learning laboratory, reading patient records, and so on. A 3-credit course should have a maximum of 6 hours per week available for out-of-class assignments. The guideline is: 2 hours of out-of-class assignments for each credit hour of class per week.

A typical full-time student takes 15 credits per semester. Applying the above guideline, this 15-credit course load is the equivalent of working full-time. For each credit, the student attends class for 1 hour each week. (The rule is usually different for lab hours, including clinical hours. In many schools, two or three lab/clinical hours are the equivalent of 1 credit hour; therefore there is less assignment time available.) Add to this number of class hours another 2 hours of homework for each class hour. Calculating the total weekly hours for a 15-credit course load, the student would spend 15 hours in class and have an additional 30 hours of home-work each week. Students with laboratory courses have even more contact hours. Over the course of a 15-week semester, a 3-credit course carries a maximum of 135 hours (45 hours of class time plus 90 hours for out of class assignments). Select carefully!

5. What happens if I assign too many hours of assignments?

Students, like all of us, are forced to make choices about how they spend their time. If you make assignments that take too many hours to complete, you lose control over which aspect of the work gets the major emphasis. Left to their own prioritization of assignments, students may not focus on areas that you consider most important.

When making reading or writing assignments, try to estimate the amount of time that it takes you to read or do the assigned work, as a relative expert in the topic. Then, double the time to arrive at an estimate of the time it will take students to complete the assignment. Remember to include term papers and studying for exams in your time estimate. Ask students who do particularly well to share with you how long it takes them to do the assignments.

6. Overall, what is most important to consider when making assignments?

Value of time spent is probably the most important factor for consideration. Ask yourself the question, "Is it worth the amount of learning time that students are spending for the value gained from the assignment?" It helps to think about the amount of time on the assignment as a proportion of student time available for the course. Similarly, your time to grade assignments (i.e., evaluate students) needs to be considered. If it takes you an hour per student to grade an assignment, it will take you 30 hours for a class of 30 students. Is that the best use of your teaching time?

Increasing the variety of thinking approaches and increasing students' repertoire of learning strategies is important. These activities enable students to examine situations from a variety of perspectives. Students need to have an increasing ability to think like a nurse and to present ideas and make decisions like a nurse.

7. What can I do to ensure that students complete the reading assignment before class?

Assign a brief task (using a 5"x 8" card) that requires analysis or synthesis of the reading to focus students on the important sections of the material. This assignment should be handed in as an "entry ticket" for class as students enter the classroom. If students do not come with the "entry ticket," they should be asked to complete it before entering the classroom. Students need to be informed ahead of time that completion of the assignment is required for entry to the classroom. You usually need to follow through with this a few times before the students believe you. Be sure to share your plans to use this strategy with other faculty and the chair/director of the program so they do not think that you are locking students out of the classroom!

8. What types of assignments can be developed to extend student thinking beyond reading?

"Notecards" can be used to generate productive discussion on assigned readings and to extend student thinking beyond the reading material. The notecard responses should include unique concerns and opinions of students. In preparing notecards, students need to record at least five complete thoughts, ideas, or reflections from the reading that they are willing to share with the group. These five points should *not* be a repetition of what is in the reading but rather should reflect what students read. These ideas are then shared in small groups, and the group summarizes and reports the questions, concerns, and issues.

9. What strategies exist to teach students to conceptualize beyond the specific content in the text?

Conceptual mapping is being used in many disciplines as a means for students to think more conceptually and to demonstrate their understanding of the relationships between concepts. Conceptual mapping is also referred to as mindmapping or brainmapping.

In nursing, conceptual mapping is often used to analyze the interrelationships between the factors influencing patient needs and intervention strategies. The major concept or client concern is written in a circle or box in the middle of the diagram (map) and then lines (like spokes on a wheel) are used to connect with other circles (or boxes) that contain related concepts. The interrelationships between the concepts are connected by lines (or dotted lines for weaker linkages). These conceptual maps can be developed in class for practice. Students can then work in groups or alone to develop the ideas and connections between the ideas. Use this group or individual work as a written assignment.

Conceptual maps are useful for the analysis of interrelationships of concepts in client situations; clinical concerns, such as immobility; professional role functions, such as research utilization; altered physiologic needs of patients; or psychosocial needs of clients in an acute care environment. The figure below illustrates a concept map for initial management of a critically injured patient.

Initial Management of the Critically Ill Patient

10. How can a nursing care plan be most effectively used as an assignment to prepare for a clinical day?

Traditional nursing care plans have been replaced by clinical pathways or similar approaches in much of the health care system. As a result, nursing education has recognized that the nursing care plan has been used as a teaching strategy to orient students to thinking like a nurse to adapt standard or textbook nursing care plans.

For many students, the nursing care plan assignment often consisted of 10 pages of preparation, which is extremely time-consuming for students to prepare and for faculty to evaluate. This assignment is more appropriately named a patient care analysis or care study. Prior to the use of clinical pathways, the nursing care plan in "real life" was not as extensive and was usually prepared to insert in a cardex file. If this type of assignment is utilized, it should be done so sparingly—no more than once a semester. If you decide to use this type of assignment, consider making it one of the major course assignments, since it requires many hours of the students' time to complete. Extensive nursing care plans should not be required for each clinical day.

The nursing care plan assignment also becomes very repetitive and does not help students learn to analyze the patient from a variety of viewpoints. As an alternative, consider assigning a different part of the care plan each week. For example, each week each student in a clinical group could analyze their patient in relation to one of Benner's[1] domains of practice; the clinical conference would focus on the clients with needs in that area.

Daily/weekly written clinical assignments should be limited to a one-page analysis or problem set which focuses on different aspects of clinical judgment with patients. Students would be encouraged to write three or four pages and then summarize the major points on the one-page write-up that is handed in. It is very important for faculty to only read the one page so that the student is forced to analyze and decide what is most important. This skill of selecting the major ideas or priorities is extremely important for the nursing practice environment.

11. How can I help students prepare for clinical learning with a preclinical written assignment?

Preclinical written assignments should focus the student on "thinking like a nurse." The students can focus on questions such as:

- What information is most important (for a nurse) to have when caring for this patient?
- What sources of information are available for planning for this patient's discharge?
- What types of interventions are typically used when caring for this type of patient?
- What nursing interventions are needed for complications in this type of postoperative situation?

These assignments should be short—one page—and should require broader reading and thinking, which would then be summarized. Short one-page assignments force the student to think through the question and select priorities, clearly an expectation of nursing practice. Also, one-page assignments are easier to grade and return to students within a short time frame while the information is still pertinent to students' learning. The skills of analyzing patient information and selecting priorities also provide a valuable lesson in clinical time management.

Notecards can also be used for clinical learning activities. Students can be asked to review the textbook materials or journal articles related to their assigned patient(s) and then generate thoughts that relate to some aspect of caring for their patients.

12. How can I use written assignments for the purpose of clinical evaluation?

Written assignments can be used in two ways:
1. To assess the student's level of preparation for the clinical experience

2. To determine the learning that occurred from the clinical experience

These assignments provide an opportunity for one-on-one exchange between the student and faculty. As such, written assignments to assess clinical preparation and post-clinical analysis can be very helpful in understanding the learner and his or her level of competence.

Consider using an assignment based upon the ideas developed by the "One Minute Manager."[4] This assignment can be used for several purposes:

• To evaluate student thinking processes
• To provide feedback about student thinking and learning related to the course
• To evaluate course activities

To use the "One Minute Manager" concept, assign a topic and allow students 60 seconds to write their thoughts about the topic. Topics can be evaluative, such as, "How do you feel about this clinical experience to date," or "What was the most important thing you learned from your clinical experience today?" This assignment poses questions with a specific focus and requests the learner's opinion. Both cognitive and affective learning can be measured in this way. These assignments should not be graded since they provide a means of one-on-one communication between faculty and student. Assignments such as these are valuable in that they provide opportunities for student reflection and assimilation of knowledge and allow faculty to identify areas where further teaching is needed.

Reflective journals can also be used for clinical evaluation purposes. Journals, also, provide an opportunity for students and faculty to communicate on an individual level. These journals can be a diary-like response to the clinical experience, or they can be directed toward topics such as Benner's domain of the helping role of the nurse. They are useful for clinical evaluation in that they identify areas in which additional teaching is needed.

13. How should written clinical assignments be graded?

Grading clinical assignments can be problematic if there are too many points attached to sections of the assignment. It is often difficult to distinguish differences between students when a 50- or 100-point scale is used for short assignments. If you wish to use a quantitative approach, consider using a grading scale of only 5, 10, or 20 points for short assignments.

For longer assignments, consider using letter grades for each section of the assignment, then adding them to arrive at the total grade. The wise faculty member will establish some qualitative criteria for an A, B, C, D, and F (plus and minus can be added for a slightly better quality or slightly less quality) *before* beginning the grading process. Sample operational definitions of the letter grades A, B, and C are:

      A: unusually outstanding analysis of ideas and their application to clinical practice
      B: good knowledge that is necessary for practice
      C: a minimum level of knowledge

For additional examples of operational definitions for letter grades, visit the following web site: http://www.criticalthinking.org/University/univclass/Profiles.nclk

Unlike a quantitative approach to grading, in which points are allocated for each section of the assignment, a qualitative approach to grading looks at the assignment as a whole, with its integration of ideas; the degree of integration provides evidence of critical thinking. However, the ability to refine a qualitative approach to grading evolves as faculty develop in their role. Therefore, faculty are cautioned of the necessity to maintain fairness and consistency in grading!

BIBLIOGRAPHY

1. Benner P: From Novice to Expert: Excellence and Power in Clinical Nursing Practice. Menlo Park, CA, Addison Wesley, 1984.
2. Blanchard DK, Johnson S, Blanchard KH: One Minute Manager. New York, William Morrow & Company, 1982.
3. Conderman GJ: Notecards promote discussion. The Teaching Professor 7:3, 5, 1993.
4. Daley BJ, et al: Concept maps: a strategy to teach and evaluate critical thinking. J Nurs Educ 38:42-47, 1999.
5. Kemp VH: Concept analysis as a strategy for promoting critical thinking. J Nurs Educ 24:382-384, 1995.
6. Romance NR, Vitale MR: Concept mapping as a tool for learning: Broadening the framework for student-centered instruction. Coll Teaching 47: 74-79, 1999.
7. Willis AS: Integrating levels of critical thinking into writing assignments for introductory psychology students. Paper presented at the Annual Meeting of the American Psychological Association, Washington DC, 1992, ED358025.

V. On the Horizon

23. THE NEW MILLENNIUM: THE ROLE OF DISTANCE EDUCATION

Carla Mueller, PhD(c), RN

1. What is meant by distance education?

Distance education is any formal approach to education in which the majority of the instruction occurs while instructors and students are at a distance from each other. Instruction (communication) may be synchronous or asynchronous. ***Asynchronous communication*** is communication that involves a delay between interaction. This occurs with correspondence courses and in some types of computer-mediated courses. In the context of computer-mediated course delivery, students and faculty are not required to be on a computer system or at a specific location at the same time (e.g., listserv, bulletin board, e-mail). ***Synchronous communication*** is communication that occurs at the same time; there is immediate student-faculty interaction. This occurs when two-way audio and/or video technology is used. In the context of computer-mediated course delivery, synchronous communication requires students and faculty to be linked through a computer and connected at the same time (e.g., chat rooms).

2. What are the current trends in distance education?

Modes of distance education delivery are undergoing rapid change, and technologies that are currently in use could soon become obsolete. Although use of correspondence courses and audio-video technologies continues, currently there is an explosion in the use of computer-mediated course delivery via the Internet. Computer-mediated course delivery is expected to become a major part of mainstream education within the next 10 years.

3. What are students' motives for studying via distance education?

Students pursue higher education via distance education for the same reasons as students who pursue higher education in a traditional on-campus setting. They want to obtain higher professional qualifications, open up new professional perspectives, increase their knowledge base, and obtain intellectual stimulation. However, the compression of time and events in daily life makes it difficult for adult students to participate in or appreciate the leisurely pace of the traditional youth-centered model of higher education to achieve a degree. The logistics of attending traditional on-campus classes has become increasingly difficulty for many adult students to manage due to work and family commitments. Students who do not live near a college or university find traveling to distant campus difficult. Students select distance education as a mode of course delivery to overcome these barriers.

4. Do students learn as well through distance education as they do through traditional education?

Research has documented the effectiveness of learning via distance education.[1,7] Students enrolled in distance education courses generally report satisfaction with the courses and with the delivery mode .[1,7] The role of faculty in distance education is one of a facilitator and evaluator rather than one of information delivery. Distance education can provide multiple representations of information, learning situated in a real-world context, and learning available at a convenient time and place. This facilitates effective learning.

5. What types of distance education are available?

Distance education may employ correspondence study, audio and/or video technologies, or computer-mediated course delivery. Three types of distance education are described in the table below.

Types of Distance Education

TYPE	DESCRIPTION
Correspondence study	Includes study via a series of printed materials, mailed or faxed between faculty and students
Audio and/or video technologies	Include course delivery via broadcast or cable television, interactive television, phone lines, and video tapes Interactive television • Allows real-time interaction between student groups • Requires students who are on-campus and at remote sites to be in specially equipped rooms • Uses broadcasts in which the video transmission may be two-way audio and video (both campus and remote sites see and hear each other) or one-way video and two-way audio (the remote sites view what is transmitted on a monitor and audio transmission occurs via a telephone line). • Two-way audio courses are transmitted via phone lines to students in multiple locations. Videotapes may be used in combination with other print materials for independent study or as file tapes of video courses for later use.
Computer-mediated course delivery	Course offering via the Internet as: • Web-based courses • Web-supported courses

Web-supported courses are those offered with a combination of traditional on-campus class meetings and meetings via the Internet. ***Web-based courses*** meet entirely via the Internet. The web site for most computer-mediated courses is password protected. Information available on the Internet includes a syllabus, reference list, lecture notes, and other information posted on multiple web pages. Computer-mediated courses may include use of a restricted listserv, using synchronous or asynchronous communication to hold discussion groups, on-line testing, and e-mail. Since synchronous communication is communication that occurs at the same time, there is immediate student-faculty interaction. In the context of computer-mediated course delivery, students and faculty are linked through a computer and connected at the same time (i.e., chat rooms). Since asynchronous communication involves a delay between interaction, students and faculty are not required to be on a computer system or at a specific location at the same time (i.e., listserv, bulletin board, e-mail).

6. Is distance education for everyone?

Distance education is *not* for everyone, but is suitable for most faculty and students. Students and faculty must believe that high-quality learning can take place without going to a traditional classroom. Faculty and students must also be willing to accept the value of facilitated learning as an advantage over the more traditional faculty-directed, lecture-based learning process. Faculty must be willing to reevaluate course design and assignments and adapt to the new course delivery mode so course objectives will be met. Learners must be self-starters with enough discipline to complete the course requirements. Many distance education programs have an accelerated pace. Students in accelerated courses who procrastinate may find that the course passes them by and that catching up is difficult, if not impossible. Learners must be able to communicate well in writing.

7. How do I develop a course for distance education?

Courses for distance education are developed differently, depending on the type of delivery mode to be used. Traditional lecture and group activities work well in interactive television courses. However, the large block of time (2-3 hours) in which these courses are offered requires faculty creativity to maintain student interest throughout the entire class period. Computer-mediated courses require a different pedagogy. In these courses, faculty move from the role of information delivery to the role of facilitator. Courses are offered in the pedagogy of computer-mediated course delivery. Faculty would be well-advised to enroll in one of these courses to assist their own course development. Campus workshops on distance education course development are also helpful. Some faculty believe that it is easier to develop a computer-mediated course from scratch rather than convert a course that they are currently teaching. Although faculty shudder at the thought of another meeting, a support group of faculty teaching distance education courses can facilitate sharing of information and successful teaching techniques.

8. I have developed a course to be delivered by distance education. Now what?

Student support services are critical to successful distance education. Traditional means of delivery of support services need to be evaluated prior to implementation of distance education courses. Because distance education students do not have ready access to traditional on-campus resources, new mechanisms for student access to services often must be developed. Arrangements must be made for phone or on-line registration (including drop/add), advising, and access to financial aid and career counselors.

The campus bookstore needs to arrange a mechanism for distance education students to obtain course textbooks and related materials. The bookstore can prepare a list of required textbooks that is accessible via the Internet or mailed to students several weeks prior to the beginning of the course. Books can then be ordered and shipped to students prior to the beginning of the semester.

Students prefer having required readings readily accessible and are willing to pay for this convenience. Relevant readings can be placed in a course handbook and sold in the campus bookstore after copyright permission has been obtained. Advances in technology now allow assigned readings to be placed on electronic reserve in the library at some universities. Electronic reserve allows students enrolled courses to have computer access to the assigned readings.

Library access is critical to enable students to complete the research for completion of assignments in distance education courses. Since distance education students may never be on campus or on campus in a limited fashion, alternative ways of obtaining library access must be developed to facilitate student access. Literature searches of databases such as MEDLINE and CINAHL are accessible via the Internet at many universities. Additionally, some universities subscribe to databases with full text articles online. Technical help in using the library via the Internet is important so that students are able to obtain necessary reference materials to complete learning activities. E-mail can facilitate communication with students who need assistance during hours the library is not open. Additional options to assist students include automated answering of frequently answered questions via the telephone, automated fax back services for delivery of library user guides, and posting of information on a library home page on the Internet.

Once support services are in place, marketing of the distance education courses can begin. It is important to inform any currently enrolled students if mode of course delivery will change. Using more than one type of notification (e.g., letter, notation in the course schedule, posting flyers at the school of nursing, and class announcements) helps to ensure that current students are aware of any changes planned in the mode of course delivery.

9. How can I be sure that the work submitted for a distance education course is actually done by the student enrolled in the course?

This is a difficult issue and is dealt with both in the traditional classroom as well as in distance education. Even in the traditional classroom setting, faculty cannot be totally certain that assignments completed at home and submitted by students were actually completed by those students. Some distance education programs use paper and pencil or computer-based testing at a secure testing site (e.g., Sylvan Learning Center) or via a proctor. Other programs administer comprehensive examinations at the home campus during a brief residency session to ensure mastery of information. Performance in clinical courses and preceptor evaluations demonstrating appropriate application of theoretical content to patient care help to ensure achievement of course outcomes.

10. What are the copyright issues related to distance education?

Faculty utilize a wealth of materials while teaching courses. Many of the materials used by faculty are protected by copyright. It is important for faculty to realize that the lack of a copyright symbol on a work does not imply that copyright is not applicable. Copyright automatically applies if the work is an original work of authorship and is fixed in a tangible form.

The Copyright Act is very specific about what types of materials can and cannot be transmitted in distance education courses. The Copyright Act makes a distinction between a *display* and a *performance*. To display is to show a copy of the work, whether directly or by means of a film, slide, television image, or to show individual images nonsequentially. A display is allowed under copyright law. A performance is to recite, render, play, dance, show images in any sequence, or to make audible accompanying sounds. The Copyright Act restricts a performance unless permission has been obtained for the performance from the copyright holder.

In traditional face-to-face teaching, nearly all displays and performances are allowed in a nonprofit educational context when activities take place in a classroom or similar location. Although faculty and students are not required to have face-to-face contact, they are required to have a simultaneous presence in a similar location. Difficulties in distance education occur when learning does not occur in a classroom or similar location and when asynchronous modes of education are used.

Late in 1998, the Digital Millennium Copyright Act was signed into law in the United States. This act could alter fundamental activities of university libraries, distance education, and web site development. Faculty would be wise to review the many copyright sites available via the Internet and contact their university copyright office prior to using material in a distance education course so as not to violate copyright law. Internet sites providing helpful information are included in the table on the next page.

Internet Sites with Copyright Information

RESOURCE	URL
The U.S. Copyright Office Home Page	http://www.loc.gov/copyright
Stanford University Library: Copyright & Fair Use	http://fairuse.stanford.edu
Georgia's Regents Guide to Understanding Copyright and Educational Fair Use	http://www.peachnet.edu/admin/legal/copyright
Distance Learning Multimedia Development Regional Center	http://www.lib.siu.edu/regional/copyright.html
The Copyright Management Center at IUPUI	www.iupui.edu/~copyinfo
Georgia Harper's Crash Course in Copyright at the University of Texas	http://www.utsystem.edu/ogc/intellectualproperty /cprtindex.htm

11. Can I teach a clinical course via distance education?

Certainly, a clinical course can be taught via distance education. Students must be linked with a preceptor or clinical instructors close to where they reside. Preceptors and clinical instructors must be thoroughly oriented to the course expectations. Faculty from the main campus can provide ongoing support to preceptors and clinical faculty through telephone conferences and e-mail. Since it is unrealistic to expect faculty at the home campus to visit students who reside at a great distance, programs can test clinical skills in a demonstration via videotapes of students' performance in a simulation, at a regional testing center, or at a brief required summer residency session. Other programs use regional faculty to make site visits and evaluate the educational appropriateness of clinical settings and evaluation students' progress.

12. How do I facilitate interaction with and among students in a distance education course?

Interaction between students is important with all learning, but is especially important in distance education. Interaction motivates and stimulates learners, clarifies course content, and facilitates socialization into the profession. Students in distance education courses are relatively autonomous learners. However, collaborative and interdependent learning activities reinforce course content and extend students' learning.

Establishing a sense of community is necessary to overcome the barriers of distance and technology found in distance education. Formation of a sense of community is facilitated by introduction of students and faculty during the first interaction. Distribution of students' and faculty pictures via a newsletter or a course home page on the Internet may help to overcome the lack of visual cues and assist students to become familiar with their peers and faculty. Learning activities should be structured to promote student interaction. Group process strategies, such as creating a safe and supportive environment, encouraging participation from all students, and acknowledging responses, can be used to facilitate interaction and enhance a sense of community. This sense of community is crucial since it facilitates socialization into the profession.

Students should be given opportunities to interact with one another outside of scheduled class times. This may be facilitated by distribution of students' phone numbers and e-mail addresses. Some computer-mediated course delivery software allows construction of a social space via a chat room. Students enrolled in courses using two-way audio and/or video technology can be given time to interact via the technology before and after class time.

Faculty must maintain office hours to facilitate communication with students. Differences in time zones where students reside must be considered when office hours are selected. Faculty should also determine whether traditional modes of contact fit the need of distance education students and make adjustments as needed. New modes of contacting faculty include e-mail, interactive video, and synchronous interaction via the Internet, using software such as NetMeeting®.

13. What challenges do faculty encounter when teaching via distance education?

- *Learning curve*. A steep learning curve exists for both faculty and students when a new mode of course delivery is implemented. A smooth transition to distance education is facilitated with advanced planning, support from a consultant, and faculty orientation to distance education pedagogy. Grants help faculty interested in developing courses for distance education by providing release time for curriculum development.
- *Course evaluation*. Both formative and summative evaluation of courses offered via distance education is important. Faculty must be willing to listen to student feedback when courses are implemented and make adjustments when needed. An informal evaluation, done in the middle of the new course, is helpful to facilitate student feedback and rectify major problems.
- *Delivery medium*. The challenges encountered are often directly related to the course delivery medium. Faculty teaching via interactive television identify the lack of eye contact with students at the distant site and the need to stay in front of a camera and microphone as major adjustments. Faculty must look at the way in which they deliver visual information. They are not able to spontaneously write on a chalkboard since students at the distant site cannot view it. Experimentation is necessary to identify what visuals display best on the television. Faculty teaching in a virtual classroom on the Internet in an asynchronous mode must prepare and post printed lectures and slides in advance. Faculty teaching computer-mediated courses using synchronous technology identify lack of eye contact and visual cues as a major adjustment.
- *Teaching workload*. Teaching loads need to be adjusted for faculty who teach courses to multiple sites and students. The load for a faculty member who teaches a class of 50 students on-campus is not the same as the load for a faculty member who teaches the same course and number of students at five different sites. Determination of faculty load should include the number of students, the number of participating sites, diversity of student populations being served, delivery technology used for course delivery, and faculty experience with distance education.
- *Testing strategies*. Testing strategies must be changed. Tests may be given via a proctor, at a secure testing site, via e-mail or the Internet, or as a take-home test, or students may be required to come to campus to take tests.
- *Student presentations*. The challenges encountered depend on the course delivery medium. Presentations by students can be videotaped and shown via interactive television, sent to students, or presented via audio only. Presentation software, such as PowerPoint® slides, can be used and even posted on the Internet; the text of a presentation can be distributed; or presentations can be given using synchronous technology such as NetMeeting®.
- *Technical support*. Technical support is critical for distance education courses to run smoothly. The type of technical support required depends on the technology used. Students taking computer-mediated courses who are not computer literate require a great deal of technical support during their first course. It is important to identify com-

puter skills necessary for successful course completion and provide avenues for students to obtain the necessary skills.

• *Compatibility of computer hardware and software*. When teaching computer-mediated courses, student and faculty computer equipment and software may not be compatible. It is important to identify the minimal computer equipment and software necessary for the course prior to registration.

• *Qualified preceptors and off-site faculty*. The lack of sufficient preceptors and off-site faculty can be a major obstacle to distance education in clinical courses. Students may be able to help identify preceptors within their geographic area. Alumni of the nursing program who have been in practice for a sufficient period of time may also be willing to serve as preceptors. Not to be overlooked are the connections which the dean or director of the nursing program may have through the American Association of Colleges of Nursing or the National League for Nursing. Course faculty may be able to identify qualified preceptors and off-site faculty through their own networking in professional nursing organizations.

• *Budgets*. Budgets need to be transformed to match the demands of distance education. Budget items change from building maintenance, heat, light, and laboratory supplies to computers, printers, software, television studios, digital cameras, scanners, fax machines, and long-distance phone calls.

Without a doubt, distance education is on the near horizon (or even here now) for many nursing programs. This mode of course delivery offers the promise of accessibility to self-directed students who, otherwise, might not be able to participate in a degree program. However, distance education is not without challenges unlike those encountered in the traditional classroom. As technology changes and faculty and students become more facile with available technology, distance education offers the promise of new avenues of teaching and learning for faculty and students.

BIBLIOGRAPHY

1. Billings DM, Bachmeier B: Teaching and learning at a distance: A review of the literature. In Allen LR (ed): Review of Research in Nursing Education. New York, National League for Nursing, 1994, pp 1-32.
2. Clark CE: Teaching and learning at a distance. In Billings DM & Halstead JA (EDS). Teaching in Nursing: a Guide for Faculty. Philadelphia, WB Saunders, 1998, pp 331-346.
3. Harasim L, Hiltz SR, Teles L, Turoff M: Learning Networks: A Field Guide to Teaching and Learning Online. Cambridge, MA, MIT Press, 1995.
4. Keegan D: Foundations of Distance Education, 3rd ed. New York, Routledge, 1996.
5. Lewis ML, Kaas MJ: Challenges of teaching graduate psychiatric-mental health nursing with distance education technologies. Arch Psychiatr Nurs 12:227-233, 1998.
6. Milstead JA, Nelson R: Preparation for an online asynchronous university doctoral course: Lessons learned. Comput Nurs 16:247-258, 1998.
7. Novotny J: Distance Learning in Nursing. New York, Springer, in press, 2000.
8. Palloff RM, Pratt K: Building Learning Communities in Cyberspace: Effective Teaching Strategies for the Online Classroom. San Francisco, Jossey-Bass, 1999.
9. Porter LR: Creating the Virtual Classroom: Distance Learning with the Internet. New York, John Wiley & Sons, 1997.
10. Willis B: Distance Education: Strategies and Tools. Englewood Cliffs, NJ, Educational Technology Publications, 1994.

24. ORGANIZATIONAL MEMBERSHIP AND POLITICAL EDUCATION: OUR FUTURE IS NOW

Elizabeth A. Mahoney, EdD, ACRN

"In unity there is strength!" This is why nurses and students of nursing must become involved, politically active members of their professional organizations. Informed membership and voting in professional and civic arenas are essential strategies to effect change. Individually and collectively, we can and must make a difference in: our patients' and their families' care, maintenance and fostering of professional practice, and influencing community and national/international health care trends. Now for some specific questions and answers.

1. What should students know about membership in professional organizations?

First, students should know why professional and student organizations were formed and their continued purposes: to protect the public and advance the profession.[1, 7] The state Nurse Practice Acts, Nursing Standards of Care, and our Code of Ethics, among other hallmarks of our profession, have been developed because of the vision and commitment of nurses who organized and collaborated to achieve common goals. Students should learn about the various categories (broad focused and specialty) and levels of nursing organizations (see tables below).[5,6]

Categories of Professional Organizations

CATEGORIES	EXAMPLES OF PROFESSIONAL ORGANIZATIONS
Broad focused	American Nurses Association (ANA)
	International Council of Nurses (ICN)
	National League for Nursing (NLN)
	National Student Nurses Association (NSNA)
Specialty	
• Clinical	Association of Operating Room Nurses (AORN)
	Nurses in AIDS Care (ANAC)
• Ethnic	National Black Nurses Association (NBNA)
	Philippine Nurses Association of America (PNAA)
• Gender	American Assembly of Men in Nursing (AAMN)
• Leadership	American Academy of Nursing (AAN)
• Religious	National Association of Prolife Nurses (NAPN)
• Role-related	American Association of Colleges of Nursing (AACN)
	American Organization of Nurse Executives (AONE)
	National Organization of Nurse Practitioner Faculty (NONPF)
Scholarship	Sigma Theta Tau International Honor Society of Nursing (STTI)

Levels and Examples of Professional Organizations

LEVELS	EXAMPLES
International	International Council of Nurses (ICN)
National	American Nurses Association (ANA)
Regional	Eastern Nursing Research Society (ENRS)
State	New York State Nurses Association (NYSNA)
Local • District • Chapter	Capital District #9 NYSNA Delta Pi Chapter, STTI

Students should know the purposes and functions of various professional associations and political organizations (e.g., political parties, League for Women Voters). Students and nurses should select their broad-focused professional associations (ANA, state and district nurses associations) and specialty organizations based on their clinical or other interests. Students should learn the requirements for membership, frequency and site of meetings, programs, process for joining, and how to become involved. Benefits of membership can include:
- Increasing the voice and revenues for professional nursing
- Educational programs
- Networking
- Journals and newsletters
- Discounts for convention registration, purchases, and certification examinations
- Tax deductions for dues and costs of meetings

Some organizations even have dues options, e.g., deferred payment, payroll deduction. Students need to learn that the value of professional membership outweighs the financial cost.

2. Why is it important that students become involved in the professional nursing organizations?

Students are the future of nursing and health care. Therefore, it is imperative that they become involved in professional nursing organizations. They are tomorrow's leaders and change agents. Without their participation the organizations will cease to be effective and eventually cease to exist. Large numbers of nurses enable professional organizations to effectively influence political and health care arenas. Fewer than 10% of the approximately two and one-half million nurses belong to their professional association. Because of low numbers, nursing organizations are increasingly challenged about whether they actually represent nurses. If they do not represent nurses, we must ask ourselves, "Who will?" and "Who will advocate for the public health?"

3. How can faculty be encouraged to become more involved in professional nursing organizations?

Ideally, faculty should not need to be encouraged to participate in professional organizations. They should be actively involved for the same reasons as students. In addition, faculty should serve as role models for students to emulate. Faculty should also be mentors to assist students in their transition to membership in the profession, understanding their rights and responsibilities, and participating in professional organizations.

Role expectations in some schools of nursing may require faculty to be members of the

ANA or the National League for Nursing (NLN) or at least one organization related to their specialty. Travel monies should be allocated among faculty for attendance at professional meetings, with priority given to those faculty actively involved at the local or state level. Programs also must support faculty by allowing time, flexibility, and creativity in scheduling so that faculty can attend meetings and still meet their work role expectations. Faculty evaluations can document and give credit for involvement in professional organizations. Faculty also can be reminded that participation as officers and committee members frequently includes travel assistance by the association. Schools and departments must remember that faculty participation in professional organizations provides advertisement for the program. Name tags state one's workplace, introductions include work roles and settings, and networking and learning enhance the knowledge base of the nursing program and educational organization.

4. How can faculty foster professional growth among students?

Faculty must be active professionally and politically to serve as role models for students.

In their initial courses, students should be introduced to the concepts of profession and professionalism: the ANA Standards of Clinical Practice (1998), with particular attention to those related to professional performance; the state Nurse Practice Act; a brief history of nursing, its organizations, and the importance of active membership; student associations, local/state/regional groups, and member meetings and topics.

Inviting a panel of officers or other representatives of nursing organizations to a class allows students to dialogue with these leaders and receive "first-hand" information. Each nursing course should have as a theme the need to know and integrate the ANA Standards and state definitions of nursing and requirements for individual practice. A course requirement of attendance at a minimum of one professional meeting each semester is a means of introducing and reinforcing the availability of and responsibility for professional participation. Announcements of upcoming meetings for various associations broaden students' knowledge about regional opportunities and offer options for participation. Faculty informing organizations of students' potential attendance at meetings enables associations to provide welcomes, orientation, introductions, and complimentary refreshments, and facilitates students' socialization process and more voluntary involvement.

5. How can faculty and students influence the profession's standards of nursing practice, nursing education, and nursing research?

Faculty and students must remember that they are accountable for adhering to the professional standards of nursing practice, education, and research. These standards are not just "nice" to know, but "need" to know and do. Therefore, as members of the profession, faculty and students can affirm or work to change these standards through becoming members in professional organization(s), reading and responding to the literature, becoming a committee member or officer, and taking a stand on issues at meetings or in writing. Opinions can be communicated to editors or committee chairs; manuscripts can be submitted for publication (what a great individual or group course project!). For example, the ANA Code of Ethics has undergone several draft revisions because members were not comfortable with suggested wording.

6. What activities can faculty and students engage in to positively influence the public's understanding of nursing and the role of the professional nurse in the health care system?

Faculty and students must educate the public about the profession of nursing and roles of the professional nurse. Starting with the basics, faculty and students must *look* professional (neatly groomed, a positive stance, clear name pins with credentials/titles) and *act* professional (in their attitude, communication, skill). Above all, they must communicate the intellectual, psychosocial, ethical, and psychomotor aspects of practice by actions as well as words. The ANA Standards of Clinical Practice (1998) and Benner's Domains of Practice[2] are excellent frameworks for describing what nurses do, e.g., assess, diagnose, set goals with patients/families, plan, implement, evaluate, help, teach and coach, monitor, ensure quality. "Administering and monitoring therapeutic interventions"[2(p.46)] most accurately conveys the critical thinking and skill that are inherent in taking a blood pressure or changing a dressing.

Faculty and students should let patients know when they are advocating for them, when their efforts have resulted in a change in the treatment plan, and when they are offering a complementary therapy. For example, B. Good, S. N., states: "Mrs. Need, I called Dr. No, told him that the pain medication was not controlling the pain, and asked for another prescription. Also, nursing research has shown that music can help decrease pain. Would you like to try this as an adjunct to the medication?" Versus: "Mrs. Need, Dr. No changed your med order. Would you like to listen to some music?"

In health care settings faculty and students can educate patients about their rights and act so those rights are respected. Other activities to increase the public's understanding of nurses' vital roles include:

- Faculty and students sponsoring and participating in health fairs
- Eliciting signatures for consumer-oriented legislation
- Providing information and health programs at schools, libraries, senior citizen, and other health centers
- Establishing clinical sites at shelters, adult and child day care programs
- Writing "letters to the editor" and health columns in newspapers
- Participating in radio and television health-focused programs
- Working with colleagues in nursing and other disciplines on- and off-campus to enhance health care
- Lobbying and working with legislators at all levels on health and other issues
- Being active in professional associations and participating in their programs

In essence, faculty and students must be visible as caring, informed, involved persons who are nurses and citizens, willing and able to make a difference.

7. What do we mean by political education?

Politics is exerting influence in decision making, especially about scarce resources, and "control over situations and events." [6(p. 9)] Therefore, political education is learning about how to exert that influence. Key components of political education are depicted in the table below.

Key Components of Political Education

COMPONENT	EXAMPLE
Understanding theories	Systems, communication, decision, change, role
Developing skills	Identification of issues, stakeholders, power figures and brokers, positions of the supporters of issues, decision making, conflict resolution, research utilization, risk taking, coalition building, team work, influencing others

The skills needed are not new to nurses; rather, many nurses simply have not used these skills to achieve political ends. Mason and Leavitt[6] emphasized the four spheres in which nurses must influence politics and policy: workplace, professional organizations, community, and government. Nurses can and must exert their collective power in these areas to protect the public and maintain quality health care.

8. How can political education be taught in the nursing curriculum?

Political education, by its definition, is or should be part of every nursing course. Many of the basic theories, skills, and professional organizations are introduced as part of the first nursing course. Political examples can be used to illustrate those theories and skills; organizational activities and positions on issues and in monitoring or initiating legislation should be part of topical discussions. Students should be encouraged to become involved in committees at school or work and be allowed input into the conduct of classes (choice of some topics, self-evaluation as part of course grade/evaluation) as means of exerting influence in the work/school environment. Faculty should work with nursing organizations to involve students in lobby days and other political action; student participation can be part of course requirements to emphasize its inherence in the professional role. Buses and other transportation can be used so that students have access to the lobbying site or local legislators' offices. Faculty advisors should work with student nurses' associations to involve them in political activities. Assignments should also include working with other community groups, e.g., senior citizens, schools, and homeless shelters, to learn about health needs, gaps in provision of care, and how to access health care resources from a consumer perspective.

9. What is faculty's role in influencing health care policy and improving the health care system?

Faculty should be directly involved as individuals and through professional and community organizations to influence health care policy and improve the health care system. Faculty should be role models, facilitators, and mentors for students. If faculty are not involved, students are less likely to be involved. Faculty disagreement with organizations' positions on issues (sometimes as "devil's advocates") can prompt vigorous debate and inform students about the various facets of the issues.

10. Is there room for student involvement in influencing health care policy and improving the health care system?

Definitely! If a purpose of education is to prepare the students for the future, students must be involved in influencing health care policy and improving the health care system. Students can work with faculty and other interested persons to learn the art of politics and how organizations function. Some examples have been presented above. In addition, as part of community nursing courses, students can work with patients and community leaders to identify and pursue needs and negotiate the political and health care systems. Some colleges have community service requirements where students learn activism at the grass roots level. States have internship programs where selected students can work in legislative and health care arenas and learn directly how systems operate. Lobby days sponsored by professional nursing organizations provide students with the opportunity to be oriented to the lobbying process, key health care issues, and rationales for nursing positions; visit legislators with experienced nurses to observe the art of meeting with staff, and ideally the legislator, and how agendas are presented; network with current and future nursing colleagues; and be socialized into another facet of the nursing role. In addition, the faculty and students' presence communicates their recognition of the value of lobbying, support for the nursing organization and its legislative platform, and a more united approach to the legislators.

11. Can faculty and students be influential in promoting and protecting the interests of nurses and nursing in the legislative, regulatory, and political arenas?

Faculty and students have a gift, by virtue of their citizenship and membership in organ-

izations, that elected officials, candidates, and promoters want—the right and responsibility to vote. Approximately 1 in 44 female voters is a nurse. What power nurses have if and
when they choose to exercise it! ANA, state, and specialty nursing organizations through
individual and collective memberships can exert great influence, as indicated by the collective action in Nursing's Agenda for Health Care Reform and against the Registered Care
Technologist (RCT) proposal.[3] Nursing's Agenda was formulated by ANA and NLN in
1991 and supported by more than 50 nursing organizations, one of the greatest collaborative
nursing efforts of recent history. Many proposals in this Agenda became part of President
Clinton's health reform platform. In 1988 physician groups developed the role and educational program for a new health care worker (RCT) for whom nurses would be accountable
but have no input into their preparation or practice. Under the leadership of professional
nursing organizations nurses united to inform physicians, legislators, and consumers about
this proposed category of provider and the potential harm to the public, the implementation
of the RCT program was successfully curtailed.

Financial and personal support of organizations' (e.g., ANA, NYSNA) Political
Action Committees (PACS) also influences outcomes of political campaigns and empha-
sizes their role as powers in elections. Professional PACs were formed to provide or
withhold financial and written support of candidates for political office. PACs hold fund-
raising events to support their activities. Many prospective and incumbent legislators for
state and federal office actively solicit ANA and state nurses association PACs for their
endorsements and use this support in their campaigns to attract more voters.
Endorsements are based on the legislators' shared values with and support of nursing and
health related issues, potential for success, political power (i.e., member or chairperson
of a major committee), among other considerations. The ANA Strategic Action Team
(N-STAT) was created as a rapid-response, grassroots effort to influence legislators and
legislation. N-STAT members are notified of pending legislation and ask to contact key
legislators, by telephone, letter, fax, e-mail, telegraph, or in-person to vote for or against
the particular proposal. Rationales and sample communication are provided for nurses to
present informed positions.

12. How can faculty and students work to protect the professional practice interests and legal rights of nurses?

Students and faculty first must acknowledge their right and responsibility to protect the
professional practice interests and legal rights of nurses as part of their commitment to society (their reason for being), as well as to the nursing profession. They need to know and
exemplify their professional nurse practice act and the standards and ethical code of nursing. These actions, clearly communicated to their patients, families, other health care
providers, and society, will promulgate a positive image about professional nursing and the
nurse advocacy role, and help society to see that supporting the professional practice of
nursing supports society's health and welfare.

Faculty and students need to understand the meaning, value, and legal implications of
their practice act, how proposed changes will affect their practice, and address the issues
accordingly.

Nurses need to unite with other nurses through professional organizations, with other
health care providers, and with actual or potential clients to form coalitions to protect the
rights of consumers and practitioners. Faculty and students need to be empowered and work
to empower others to maintain standards and participate in changes that will advance the
well-being of society and the profession. They need to apply their skills in using the nursing process and critical thinking to the professional and political arenas—the problem-
solving, decision-making processes are the same.

13. What should students know about collective bargaining in the nursing workplace?

Students need to know the definition, history, process, issues, and current relevance of collective bargaining, especially the need for and value of being represented by a professional organization in contrast to a trade or non-nursing agent, and its relationship to organizational governance. They need to know the purpose, history, restructuring of the American Nurses Association, and ways of organizing. They also need to learn and use negotiation skills in the workplace to establish and maintain an environment that is conducive to professional practice and safe patient care.

Nursing is at a critical point in its collective bargaining history. Trade unions (e.g., 1199; Teamsters; and other non-nursing unions, such as teachers' unions) are experiencing decreases in numbers and the need to increase revenues and, therefore, are looking for new markets. Many nurses work in very stressful environments (high patient acuity, understaffing, more demands and fewer resources), with compromised quality of care and greater risk for error. These conditions are making nurses receptive to external support to promote change in the workplace (to restore quality care) and vulnerable to outside influences. Nurses best know professional values and issues. State nurses associations have been effective bargaining agents for nurses but do not have the resources that many trade unions possess and may not be able to "wine and dine" nurses to recruit them. Many trade unions use professional jargon to sound like nursing organizations in their invitations to nurses to join their ranks. The major issue in all of this is who represents nurses—the professional association (ANA and state nurses associations) or trade unions, whose focus is on numbers and money, regardless of the discipline and its values. If nurses do not belong to their professional association, nurses may not represent nurses at the bargaining table or in the International Council of Nurses. Nurses must become knowledgeable about the differences between the professional and trade organizations; be aware that professional dues fund the development and revision of nursing standards; and be aware of practice, educational, legislative, and economic programs that enhance patient care, public welfare, and nursing interests. The recent restructuring of the ANA resulted in streamlining organizational units to fund key projects and areas of concern and to strengthen the economic and general welfare program that includes collective bargaining.

14. Is there a role for faculty and students in lobbying their elected officials? If so, what is it?

As mentioned earlier, faculty and students definitely have a role in lobbying their elected officials. As voters they have access to and bargaining power with persons in or aspiring to political office. Faculty and students need to exercise that power for the public and profession's welfare. Roles for faculty include:
- Write, call, and visit their elected representatives
- Participate in lobby days
- Circulate and sign petitions
- Work in political campaigns
- Join district nursing association's legislative committees.

Faculty and students must communicate their understanding of the issues relevant to consumers and specific to the profession. A review of state nurses associations' legislative agendas can indicate and support the scope of issues, and demonstrate that nurses' concerns are not self-serving but have the public welfare as their focus.

In summary, faculty, students, and all nurses need to be politically active in the workplace, professional organizations, community, and government. Preparation for these roles must be as integral to the nursing curriculum as administering and monitoring medication effects for nurses' and patients' safety and well-being.

BIBLIOGRAPHY

1. American Nurses Association: American Nurses Association Bylaws, Washington, DC, 1999.
2. Benner P: From Novice to Expert. Menlo Park, CA, Addison-Wesley, 1984.
3. Catalano JT: Contemporary Professional Nursing, Philadelphia, FA Davis, 1996.
4. Kalisch PA, Kalisch BJ: The Advance of American Nursing, 3rd ed. Philadelphia, Lippincott, 1995.
5. Kelly LY, Joel LA: The Nursing Experience: Trends, Challenges, and Transitions, 3rd ed. New York, McGraw-Hill, 1996.
6. Mason DJ, Leavitt JK: Policy and Politics in Nursing and Health Care, 3rd ed. Philadelphia, WB Saunders, 1998.
7. New York State Nurses Association: Functions and Structure. Guilderland, NY, 1999.
8. Nunnery RK: Advancing Your Career: Concepts of Professional Nursing, Philadelphia, FA Davis, 1997.
9. Schwirian PM: Professionalization of Nursing, 3rd ed. Philadelphia, Lippincott, 1998.

VI. Pulling It All Together

25. LESSONS LEARNED: PERSPECTIVES FROM A NEW FACULTY MEMBER

Jenny Radsma, MN, RN

1. I have always practiced clinical nursing. This is my first experience as a faculty member. I am both excited and apprehensive about this new avenue in my career. Is this "normal?"

Experiencing a full range of emotions is all part of the anticipation and transition you are making from a nurse clinician to that of a nurse educator. Such emotions are likely to continue for a time, particularly as you assimilate the knowledge, skills, and values that are a part of your new role within a new setting among a new reference group.

2. What should I expect as I make the transition from clinical practice to nursing education?

You have chosen a very dynamic career path, and you can expect a great deal from it. On any given day you can expect to feel challenged, stimulated, overwhelmed, overextended, stressed, anxious, and even frustrated. In contrast, you will also have experiences in which you feel competent, confident, humbled, and ultimately, very rewarded. Recognizing the difference you can make in the lives of students and their beginning socialization to nursing offsets any drawbacks and anxieties you may feel initially.

3. Tell me about some of the stressors I can expect to encounter as a new faculty member.

The first two to three years (and some would even say the first five years) are typically rather stressful for new faculty. With each successive year, however, your competence increases proportionately to the growth of your knowledge and skill as a teacher.

From the onset, you will be confronted with meeting criteria for reappointment, tenure, and promotion. For most colleges, this means that faculty are required to demonstrate their growing competence in the areas of teaching, service, practice, and scholarship. Reappointment is often an annual occurrence until the faculty member is eligible to apply for tenure and/or promotion. (Some colleges and universities have multi-year probationary appointments.) The criteria and process for reappointment, tenure, and promotion, as well the time lines, vary from campus to campus. Lack of feedback in some environments can pose an additional stressor, and this can also be perceived as a lack of support.

Learning to teach while teaching to learn is demanding and time-consuming. Achieving a balance between the amount and quality of work within limited time frames is also stressful, particularly if you are involved in clinical and didactic instruction. The feeling of role stress is often compounded by departmental, campus, or community obligations. Meeting the needs of work and personal life also contributes to the strain of adapting to this new role.[1,2,6,7] Furthermore, you may experience reality shock, wherein the ideals you hold conflict with the realities of your experience.

4. What are the rewards that help to offset the stressors?

Most notably, nursing faculty have the good fortune to enjoy a great deal of autonomy, which requires one to enjoy working as a self-directed professional with limited
supervision. Working on your scholarly pursuits in the context of your position is both
stimulating and gratifying. Furthermore, a 9-month contract, or even a 12-month contract with summers "off," allows you the time needed to accomplish and promote these
pursuits.

Interacting with students and colleagues, or debating with some of the brightest people within your own or another discipline, is intellectually and professionally stimulating. The influence that you have upon your students and the impact they have upon your
growth and development is ultimately why we seek to become nursing educators.

5. Where should I focus my efforts when I begin my new role as an educator?

Arrange a meeting with your dean as soon as possible to discuss, among other things,
your workload. The sooner you are aware of your responsibilities, the sooner you can begin
to plan and prepare for your upcoming workload assignment.

**6. I was told that I will be responsible for a 12-credit teaching load. How do I put this
into perspective within my work week?**

You will want to know what your exact responsibilities are in relation to your
assigned credits hours. In most cases, a different ratio of credits to contact hours is used
for didactic versus clinical or laboratory teaching responsibilities. For example, a 1:1
ratio means that the faculty is given one workload credit for every hour of instruction,
whereas a 3:1 ratio entails three hours of instruction for every workload credit assigned.
In some institutions, credits may be allotted for activities such as course development,
conducting research, or grant writing. In some cases, nontraditional forms of instruction
such as distance learning courses are also awarded additional workload credits. (More on
this in Chapter 3, "The Role of Faculty within the College or University.")

7. What are my overall responsibilities for courses in which I am the sole teacher?

While the expectations may vary from campus to campus, essentially you are responsible for conducting all the activities, from start to finish, inherent in a course offering.
This usually includes preparing the course outline, coordinating any clinical experiences,
arranging guest speakers, preparing course examinations, providing students with feedback, and ensuring that the content taught is congruent with the course objectives. (Turn
to Chapter 4, "Classroom Teaching," for more on this.)

Talk to your dean about meeting curriculum objectives and program outcomes. If you
are responsible for covering specific content in your class, you want to ensure that is
incorporated into the course. Moreover, you will want to learn how your course "fits" into
the total curriculum.

While you may bear primary responsibility for an assigned course, remember that
your program will have many resources with which to assist you. A previous course syllabus is a good place to start. Discussion with a faculty member who may have taught the
course, or reviewing the course textbook with its instructional aides, will provide you
with a great deal of information.

8. How much time is "enough" when it comes to classroom preparation?

New faculty tend to overprepare for their classroom teaching, sometimes at the
expense of other responsibilities and interests, so be prepared for feeling overwhelmed, at
least in the beginning. Research indicates that new teachers average between 2½–4 hours
preparing for every hour in the classroom. Exemplary new faculty are able to bring this

preparation time to $1\frac{1}{2}$ hours per classroom hour, usually by the third or fourth semesters of instruction.[1]

9. What else do I need to be aware of in relation to my teaching role?

Your teaching role will occupy most of your time during your first year as a nursing educator. While none of the individual components inherent in your teaching role is necessarily difficult (e.g., exam preparation or student evaluation), combined they comprise a process that requires time to master. Your approach to, and philosophy of, teaching and learning will guide you to instill the quality you want within your teaching. Be sure to avail yourself of any teacher effectiveness resources that are available to you through your campus.

10. What can I do to enhance my skills as an educator?

Talk about teaching, whether with colleagues in your department, on your campus, or elsewhere within your professional network. Attend conferences that address concerns common to nursing educators and seek out teacher effectiveness resources within your campus.

Pay attention to any formal or informal feedback, whether written student evaluations, or verbal feedback from your peers. If you have any concerns about these evaluations, ask your dean or mentor to help you put them into perspective.

11. How important is it to teach the same courses from year to year?

Each time you teach a new course, you can anticipate spending a great deal of time planning and preparing for the course. You may be knowledgeable about the content required for a course, but mastery within the teaching role takes time. Consistency of your teaching load, therefore, is a definite asset for enhancing your success. Familiarity with content, improved organization, and refinement of teaching strategies all allow you to improve your teaching skill.

12. Will I need to negotiate consistency of my teaching load?

Hopefully, your dean is aware of how to assign a teaching load that is congruent with the needs of novice faculty. However, it is important for you to discuss your needs with your dean so that a balance can be achieved between your needs as a novice educator and the needs of the program.

13. What do I need to know about student evaluation?

Student evaluation is a two-way process: your evaluation of students and their evaluation of you. As the course or clinical instructor, you will evaluate students through written work, examinations, or presentations, as well as through clinical performance evaluations. Chapter 5 (Clinical Teaching), Chapter 16 (Student Evaluation), Chapter 21 (Teaching and Evaluating Critical Thinking), and Chapter 22 (Developing Written Assignments) include valuable insights on evaluating students.

Upon the conclusion of a course, students usually evaluate faculty. Student evaluation of faculty should be done using a standardized measure that ensures students' anonymity. Some schools use commercial instruments, whereas other schools develop their own instruments. Whether developed externally or internally, instruments should have good validity and reliability.

New faculty have a tendency to personalize students' evaluations of their teaching. Since teaching expertise develops over time, evaluations of faculty during the first few semesters may not be as positive as the faculty member would like. Moreover, the faculty member might be embarrassed, particularly if the evaluations are read by the dean or others. However, it is important that faculty recognize that developing teaching expertise is an evolutionary process, and that they view students' evaluations of their teaching from a professional, rather than a personal, perspective. Often, faculty are devastated when students' evaluations contain less than positive ratings or comments. Obviously, if the entire class provides negative feedback, you will want to discuss this with your dean and identify root causes, if possible. While not discrediting negative student feedback, faculty should not allow such feedback to dominate their thoughts and drain their initiative. Try to remember those great positive comments, too!

14. What do I need to know about peer evaluation?

Practices vary from campus to campus. However, peer evaluation is often an annual event during which you will be evaluated by your campus peers. Peer evaluation varies in scope from a classroom or clinical observation to evaluation of your overall teaching, service, and scholarship activities. Ask your dean or mentor about the criteria used so that you can include them as a part of your 5-year plan for professional development.

15. It seems as though my dean plays a pivotal role to my success as an educator. Is this an accurate perception?

Yes. It is important for you to meet with your dean as soon as possible after signing your contract, for several reasons. First, discuss your workload and responsibilities for the upcoming semester. Second, let your dean know that you would like to begin to map out a 5-year career path that will assist you to achieve success in your role. This plan should also reflect your goals, expectations, and scholarly interests.

Support and feedback are also important for new faculty, and your dean will be instrumental in fostering this. The dean can also be instrumental in pairing new faculty with an experienced faculty member for the purpose of mentorship. (Turn to Chapter 11, "Mentoring New Faculty", for great insights about mentoring.)

16. Is there anything in particular that I should expect from an orientation?

Orientation is a very important means for you to become introduced to people as well as to the culture of your campus and department. While campuses differ in the orientation programs they offer, you will want to become familiar with some campus and department specifics. In particular, ensure that you have an opportunity to review the mission of the institution, the organizational structure, the geographic layout of the campus, pay and benefits, faculty governance, the library, and other resources available to faculty.

17. What in particular should I expect from an orientation to the nursing department?

Here are some starting points:
- Knowledge about the history, philosophy, conceptual framework, and an overview of how the program is sequenced
- Faculty and staff composition of the department. For example, how many faculty are employed by the department? What are their specialities and areas of interest? How many and what types of staff are employed by the department? What are their responsibilities?
- Student body. How many students are in each class? What is the number of graduates annually? What are the NCLEX success rates? How many students can you expect in the classes or clinical groups you teach?
- Clarify the expectations for promotion and tenure, since plotting your way toward that goal begins *now* as you begin your new role.
- Introductions to your colleagues and department staff are also very important.

18. Do I have any legal concerns as a faculty member that are different from my role in clinical practice?

As with a clinical practice position, you must be licensed in your state and in good standing with the state board of nursing. As an educator, you are responsible for providing instruction that is consistent with current practice standards, and of course, adherence to the nurse practice act. Remember, too, that you are obligated to maintain whatever certifications you held upon employment. Additional legal (and ethical) issues are discussed in Chapter 13.

19. Is there anything in particular that I can do to seek out the support of my colleagues?

Support from your colleagues can assist you in a variety of ways, whether in teaching, scholarship, grant writing, or facilitating your socialization to the campus or community. If the support you require is slow to materialize, take some initiative yourself. Seek out your experienced colleagues. Glean what you can from their knowledge, skills, and resources. As you get to know your peers, let them know how they might assist you.

Be sure to get to know your campus colleagues as well, since they, too, can be an invaluable source of support. Sharing your experiences with other new faculty can also help you to "normalize" your experiences and perceptions.

20. What can I expect from the university in terms of professional development?

This is a good question to ask during your orientation. Institutions vary in terms of their faculty development policies, but you will want to know early on what is available, and what you must do to access such support. You will also want to know what, if any, support is available to you for continuing your education, especially if you are considering doctoral studies.

21. Like many other nurses, I expect a lot of myself, especially with new undertakings. Is there any wisdom or advice that I can use to help cope?

Most of the wisdom you need you have within yourself. However, it always bears repeating. Follow what you learned as a child: eat properly, get enough sleep, exercise regularly, spend time with friends and family, and cultivate interests outside of your work.

Other suggestions include:

- Distinguish between essential and "backburner" priorities.
- Set goals for yourself that are realistic and achievable within the limits of your time.
- Organize your time in a way that works for you, for example, "to do" lists; be sure to leave room in your day for the unforeseen; use a calendar to plan your day, week, semester, and year.
- Recognize when and where you work best. For example, work at home or in the library if this means uninterrupted time for classroom preparation.
- Protect the time you need to work *without* interruption. Be sure that students are aware of your office hours, or have them meet with you by appointment rather than dropping in at a time when you may be working productively.
- Intersperse your work with whatever makes you feel good. Indulge yourself with spontaneous things like a warm bath or going to a movie. Participate in activities throughout the semester that require planning, such as tickets to a concert or a weekend away.
- Do not minimize the importance of the social support from others whether on or off campus.[9]

BIBLIOGRAPHY

1. Boice R: New faculty as teachers. J Higher Educ 62:150-173, 1991.
2. Crepeau EB, Thibodaux L, Parham D: Academic juggling act: Beginning and sustaining an academic career. Am J Occup Ther 53:25-30, 1999.
3. Genrich S J, Pappas A: Retooling faculty orientation. J Prof Nurs 13:84-89, 1997.
4. Hodges LC, Poteet GW: The first 5 years after the dissertation. J Prof Nurs 8:143-147, 1992.
5. Magnussen L: Ensuring success: The faculty development plan. Nurse Educ 22:30-33, 1997.
6. Mobily PR: An examination of role strain for university nurse faculty and its relation to socialization experiences and personal characteristics. J Nurs Educ 30:73-80, 1991.
7. Oermann MH: Work-related stress of clinical nursing faculty. J Nurs Educ 37:302-304, 1998.
8. Oermann MH: Role strain of clinical nursing faculty. J Prof Nurs 14:329-334, 1998.
9. Sorcinelli MD: New and junior faculty stress: Research and responses. New Directions for Teaching and Learning 50:27-37, 1992.

26. BEEN THERE, DONE THAT: CASE STUDIES IN NURSING EDUCATION

This final chapter is one of case studies culled from the collective experiences of chapter authors. All names have been changed and some situations have been fictionalized to maintain anonymity. There is, however, enough truth remaining in these case studies to allow others to benefit from our collective experiences. Case studies are based upon lived experiences of many of our nurse faculty authors. The reader should not assume that any particular case study was contributed by the author who wrote a chapter related to the case study's content.

CASE 1: Maintaining Student Standards

Unfolding of Events

Mitzi, 48 years old, was a second semester nursing student who was sponsored by a state agency. She entered the nursing program for retraining following repetitive motion injuries in a previous job. She also suffered from post-traumatic stress disorder from a previous history of trauma. While taking pre-nursing courses, she requested, and received, double time for all exams. Additionally, Mitzi was permitted to take all exams in a private room in the learning center. During the first semester of nursing courses, the faculty permitted Mitzi to continue this testing routine.

At the beginning of the second semester, the faculty questioned the advisability of continuing the testing accommodations. They consulted with the college disabilities coordinator who verified that Mitzi had no disabilities that required accommodations. The disabilities coordinator stated that any accommodations would be at the faculty's discretion and that Mitzi would not be permitted extra time for taking the NCLEX.

Faculty believed that a written contract was needed to outline academic expectations for Mitzi. The contract would state specifically how much time would be allowed for exams and the location in which they would be administered. Mitzi was adamantly opposed to the idea of a contract. She insisted on a mediation session with a counselor and faculty.

Resolution

The mediation session was tense; Mitzi was hostile and accused faculty of being cold and unfeeling. With the counselor's help, Mitzi was able to review the contract. The contract gradually decreased the time permitted for each exam and assimilated Mitzi back into the classroom setting for her exams over a two-semester time period. By her last semester, Mitzi would be taking exams in the normal allotted time and in a regular classroom with her classmates. Faculty believed that requiring Mitzi to take exams in the normal allotted time and in a regular classroom environment would better prepare her to take NCLEX under expected circumstances.

Comments

The Americans with Disabilities Act, as applied to higher education, was designed to ensure equal access to educational opportunities for individuals with documented disabilities. As is sometimes the case, students attempt to gain accommodations for conditions that are not protected by the Act. Perhaps in this student's case, low self-esteem and lack of confidence contributed to her perception that she needed additional support. Faculty were wise in recognizing the need to maintain academic standards, while at the same time demonstrating sensitivity to the student's perceived needs. Their gradual "weaning" of Mitzi from additional test-taking time and solitude to the normal test-taking conditions to better prepare her for NCLEX was likely in the student's best interests and necessary to preserve the academic standards of the program.

CASE 2: Tenure Track: Making Time for Research and Scholarship

Unfolding of Events

As a new faculty member, Meredith realized that there were many role expectations, but she was not sure how to go about setting priorities and long-term plans. She knew that in 5 years she would be reviewed for tenure, and would need evidence of at least two refereed publications, university and community service, and teaching excellence. She found herself devoting all of her time to teaching, which she enjoyed but also found demanding. She researched the topics for classroom presentations and began to devote many extra hours to the delivery of content. Her lectures were enhanced with PowerPoint presentations and her clinical conferences included self-developed case studies. Preparation of test questions was a new area, and Meredith realized that she needed to learn a great deal about test mapping and item construction. Feedback from students was positive, but Meredith knew that this was only a part of role expectation.

In addition to classroom and clinical instruction, Meredith was also responsible for student advisement and had been assigned to the School of Nursing Curriculum Committee. Additionally, she was expected to participate in course team meetings. When was she going to be able to concentrate on her research and service? Teaching, though important, was just not going to be enough. After her first year in the position, Meredith met with the chair of the department and shared her concern.

Resolution

Following the discussion and review of criteria for tenure, the chair suggested that Meredith might benefit from a mentor. A seasoned faculty member would be assigned to work closely with Meredith during the next few years. Meredith and the program chair also worked out a 3-year plan with goals in each of the areas: teaching, service, and scholarship. They also discussed ways in which projects could be distributed to include summers. Meredith planned to concentrate on teaching and service goals during the academic part of the year, and become immersed in her research in the summer. The multi-year plan was reassuring for Meredith since she could stop feeling guilty about what she wasn't doing. She also knew that she was "chipping" away at all areas and would have time to reach goals by the time of her tenure review.

Comments

The lack of structure in the academic role may be welcomed by some individuals but difficult for others. For faculty who have difficulty setting limits and goals, all of their time will be pulled into teaching or service, leaving little room for research and scholarship. Depending on the individual's work style, some faculty members find it helpful to work with another person who complements their style. Scheduling regular times and days for research can provide structure, especially when getting started.

CASE 3: How and Where Do I Get Started on Research and Scholarship?

Unfolding of Events

Though Jennifer has held staff and supervisory positions in clinical practice, this is her first faculty appointment. Her master's degree had a clinical nurse specialist focus in adult health and her practice areas were concentrated on caregiver issues related to HIV/AIDS. As part of her master's degree, Jennifer completed a group research project dealing with pain management.

In addition to her teaching and service responsibilities, Jennifer is anxious to begin submitting articles for publication, but she is not sure how to begin. Jennifer understands that she should focus on referred journals; however, she also realizes that such manuscripts should be grounded in research. She is concerned about how much time will be needed to conduct research and publish, and wonders if some activities should be done ahead of others, given the time constraints. Jennifer is aware that she tends to procrastinate and has difficulty getting started. When working alone, she gets distracted easily and realizes that part of the problem may be not knowing how to develop a research agenda for herself.

Resolution

Jennifer met with her mentor, a successful nurse researcher. They started by examining Jennifer's areas of strength and knowledge. It was apparent that Jennifer was very familiar with quantitative research designs and instrument development. They discussed the importance of working in an area that was of interest to Jennifer and also would contribute to either her clinical practice or area of teaching. All of this would eventually tie into an area of expertise for Jennifer. They decided on an approach that would help to launch Jennifer's research plan.

Jennifer would begin to work with another faculty member, Carrie. Carrie was a young researcher who had one publication based on her exploratory research on coping. When Jennifer and Carrie met, they found an immediate match. Jennifer's knowledge of research design and measurement could fit with any topic and was just the area in which Carrie felt "shaky." As they began to discuss coping, Jennifer could easily apply the concept to persons with AIDS and AIDS caregivers, while Carrie was interested in any chronic, debilitating illness. They also learned that their style of working was complementary. Jennifer welcomed the "let's get started and get our ideas down" approach that Carrie used. Soon the two otherwise unlikely young researchers were targeting funding sources and setting up files branching in a variety of directions.

Comments

Researchers can find common areas in broad concepts, research design, and working style. Working with a colleague can also help young researchers with the most important beginning steps. By discussing and thinking creatively, research problems can take shape more quickly in a dialogue when compared to working alone. For Jennifer, working with another person also provided structure and discipline, which she found helpful.

CASE 4: A Student Who Abused Alcohol and Drugs

Unfolding of Events

Gerald, 45 years old, was a student in the evening undergraduate nursing program. While he was enrolled in the nursing program, he held a full-time job in the computer industry. His use of alcohol was noted by faculty on several occasions, when he arrived with the odor of alcohol on his breath. However, because he was not in possession of alcohol at the time, he did not violate the student alcohol policy. Over the next year, Gerald's repeated use of alcohol was noted on several occasions outside of class. His grades began to suffer, and faculty discussed the situation with him, advising him to seek treatment. Several months later, when he was assigned to the health department, he disappeared for a period of time during the clinical day. An hour later, Gerald reappeared, attempted to borrow money from health department staff, and, when unsuccessful, left. Later that day, Gerald reappeared, this time agitated and disoriented. The field supervisor sent him home. Unfortunately, the instructor was at another clinical site and was not informed of the incident until 1 week later. Upon learning of the incident, the instructor confronted Gerald, who admitted to taking hydrocodone bitartrate and acetaminophen (Vicodan), which he said had been prescribed by his physician for a chronic injury. Gerald's clinical performance did not meet expected standards and he received a failing grade for the course. Disciplinary charges were not filed since the instructor had not observed the behavior directly and an entire week had elapsed until she was informed. It was believed that there was insufficient documentation of the incident for the school to prevail in a disciplinary proceeding. Since he was not permitted to continue in the program until he repeated the course, Gerald did not enroll for the following semester. Several months later, the chairperson of the nursing program received a telephone call from the district attorney who advised her that Gerald had been arrested for a misdemeanor—possession of heroin. Gerald was notified that he would not be permitted to enroll in any nursing courses until the outcome of the arrest was known. Nothing further was heard from or about Gerald until 1 year later when the chairperson was again notified by the district attorney of a second arrest for possession of heroin. At that time, the first arrest had not been resolved. Gerald was now facing trial on both arrests. However, he made no attempt to return to the college, even though he had only two courses to complete to graduate.

Resolution

Gerald entered a guilty plea on both counts of possession and agreed, as part of the plea, to withdraw from the nursing program.

Comments

While the notion of a student who actively abuses alcohol and heroin is frightening, academic administrators must proceed cautiously. The school has the obligation to protect the health and welfare of all patients while being careful not to violate the rights of the student. Pursuit of a college education and a career in one's chosen profession is a property right that cannot be taken away indiscriminately. Although there were suspicions that Gerald had been under the influence of a prescription drug during the health department clinical, there was insufficient documentation to proceed with disciplinary charges. Once Gerald pleaded guilty to possession of heroin on two separate occasions, even though the incidents occurred off campus when Gerald was not in school, he was in direct violation of the college's drug and alcohol abuse policy. At this point, the college had sufficient documentation to dismiss Gerald from the nursing program. Since Gerald agreed to withdraw from the program, disciplinary charges were not filed.

CASE 5: Student Falsification of the Clinical Record

Unfolding of Events

Karen, a senior nursing student, was enrolled in her last nursing course prior to graduation. She was assigned to care for several patients on a step-down unit of a busy medical center. During pre-conference that morning, the instructor reviewed students' patient care plans and ascertained that they would begin their patient care by completing a nursing assessment on each patient, according to hospital protocol. A short time later, the instructor passed by the room of Karen's patient, noting that the patient was eating breakfast. Karen was not in the room. When the instructor reviewed the patient's chart, she noted that Karen had already completed the nursing assessment checklist, indicating that the assessment had been completed. Vital signs were recorded, as was an assessment of the cardiovascular and respiratory systems, abdomen, and extremities. Concerned that not enough time had elapsed for the student to complete the assessment, the instructor returned to the patient's room. The patient, an alert and oriented priest, told the instructor that Karen had visited him briefly, taking his blood pressure, pulse, and temperature, and helped set up his breakfast tray. When asked specifically by the instructor whether Karen had examined his heart, lungs, abdomen, and extremities, the priest stated that she had not. The instructor then left the room, called Karen aside, and asked her whether she had completed the assessment that she had charted. Karen stated that she had completed the entire assessment. When confronted with the instructor's information provided by the priest, Karen denied having falsified the record. The instructor dismissed Karen from the clinical area immediately, informed the nurse manager of the incident, and obtained a written statement from the patient. Upon returning to the college, the instructor notified the chairperson of the nursing program. The instructor filed disciplinary charges against Karen, alleging that she had practiced nursing fraudulently, a violation of the student clinical conduct code.

Resolution

In accordance with the policy, charges were presented to Karen in writing and a hearing was scheduled. Karen had legal representation at the hearing. The committee that heard the charges determined that Karen had falsified the patient's record and recommended dismissal from the course. The chairperson upheld the recommendation and notified Karen that she was dismissed from the course and would receive a failing grade. Karen appealed the decision of the chairperson and lost the appeal. She received a failing grade from the course and did not graduate.

Comments

Karen's behavior had serious implications for her career as a nurse. Honesty and integrity in one's conduct are paramount to professional nursing practice. Fortunately, the college had a student clinical conduct policy that addressed fraudulent practice. Karen's rights were protected through due process proceedings. While the incident was unfortunate, the college had a mechanism in place to deal fairly with such conduct.

CASE 6: Student with a Learning Disability

Melanie encountered her first difficulty with nursing courses in her junior year when she failed a nonclinical nursing course. As per college policy, the student was permitted to repeat the course, which she did successfully. The following year, while enrolled in a junior-level medical-surgical nursing course, Melanie again experienced difficulty. The instructor reported that Melanie was unable to function safely in the clinical area. Melanie had difficulty on several occasions with matching medication labels to the medication order. Additionally, she transposed numbers when reading the prescribed dosage. On two occasions, the instructor had intercepted what would have been medication errors had Melanie been permitted to administer the drugs. Moreover, the instructor reported that Melanie had acted impulsively, turning off a medication infusion pump when it alarmed. Melanie did not inform anyone that she had turned off the pump. When the instructor discussed the problems with Melanie, she claimed that she was learning disabled and would require special accommodations to function safely in the clinical area. The instructor contacted the college's Coordinator for Persons with Disabilities, who met with Melanie and confirmed that special accommodations were warranted. The question that arose was, "What accommodations were reasonable, given the demands of clinical nursing practice?"

The student met with a disabilities therapist, at her own expense, who recommended that Melanie be given additional time to complete clinical assignments. The student requested, and was granted, an additional hour for each clinical day as well as several additional weeks to complete the course. The instructor and student arrived at the clinical area an hour early each clinical day. Melanie used that time to review her patient's medications and treatment plan, and to familiarize herself with equipment and the patient's medical record. Concerned about the learning needs of other students in the clinical group and the need for close supervision of Melanie, the college assigned a second clinical instructor to assist the primary instructor.

Resolution

Working one-on-one with a clinical instructor, adding an additional hour to the clinical day, and extending the clinical experience by 6 weeks, Melanie was able to successfully meet all clinical objectives. The instructor who added an hour to her clinical day did so without additional compensation. However, the instructor was compensated by the student for the additional 6 weeks needed to complete the course. The student completed the remainder of the program without any accommodations, graduated, passed NCLEX, and is employed as a registered nurse.

Comments

The learning-disabled student who experiences difficulty with numbers and letters presents a unique challenge to clinical faculty. While reasonable accommodations are warranted, faculty must be cognizant of the need for the student to meet the requirements for safe patient care. Case law has established that reasonable accommodations do not necessitate a lowering of academic standards. Students who pursue practice professions, such as nursing, must demonstrate the ability to practice safely. While the student may complete the nursing program and pass NCLEX with reasonable accommodations, the issue remains about the individual's ability to function safely and effectively as a registered nurse, given today's high-acuity, fast-paced health care arena.

CASE 7: Academic Dishonesty

Unfolding of Events

The instructor assigned a term paper as part of the requirements for completion of a junior-level nursing course. After reading several papers, the instructor came upon a paper that sounded surprisingly similar to a paper that had been submitted by another student. Upon careful examination, the instructor determined that the two papers were exactly the same. The instructor confronted each student individually, informing the students that their papers were exactly the same. Initially, both students denied having copied each other's paper. The instructor then reviewed with each student the college policy on academic dishonesty. One student vehemently denied any involvement in academic dishonesty. Several days later the other student admitted to the instructor that she had copied the other student's paper with that student's permission. Ultimately, the second student admitted that she had given her friend permission to copy her paper.

Resolution

Both students received a grade of F on the paper. Because of the percentage allocation of the paper toward the final course grade, both students failed the course. Ultimately, both students withdrew from the nursing program.

Comment

Academic dishonesty must not be tolerated for any student. The school's policy for academic dishonesty was appropriately implemented by the instructor.

CASE 8: Using a Case Study to Teach in the LRC

Module for Chest Tube Drainage

The nursing learning resource center (LRC) is an arena that focuses on application of theoretical material in a simulated setting. As such, students have the opportunity to apply new information in a controlled situation with faculty supervision and feedback. Often, the teaching method used in the LRC is demonstration by the instructor with return demonstrations by students. However, faculty are also challenged to develop cognitive skills as well as psychomotor skills in this setting. This case study offers the opportunity to develop critical thinking and psychomotor skills in the LRC.

Case Study Scenario

Mr. Davidson is a trauma patient following a severe motorcycle crash. The nurse's assessment reveals a respiratory rate of 24, diminished breath sounds on the left side and no breath sounds on the right side, shallow respirations with minimal thoracic excursion, and oxygen saturation by pulse oximetry of 90% on room air. A chest tube was placed by the ER MD and a chest tube drainage system was placed to remove a pneumohemothorax on the right side of his lung.

Case Study Questions and Activities

- What is the definition of a pneumohemothorax?

- Assess the location of the chest tube on the mannequin. Note the intercostal space where the chest tube is inserted.

- Is the dressing on the chest tube sites safely secured?

- What is the problem with not maintaining a dry occlusive dressing at all times?

- For this patient with chest tubes connected to a water seal drainage unit, explain the significance of the following assessment findings and the appropriate nursing actions.

    - The fluid level in the water seal drainage unit fluctuates with each respiration.
    Significance: An effective water seal requires at least 2 cm of water throughout inspiration and expiration. The water seal acts as a one-way valve, allowing air out of the chest but not back in. Tidaling is the fluctuation of this fluid column normally seen with inspiration and expiration. A rise is seen with inspiration and a fall with expiration.
    Nursing action: Observe the normal presence of tidaling. If it is not present the tube may be clogged with a clot or lung tissue. Notify the physician if any abnormality is discovered.

    - Continuous bubbling occurs in the water seal drainage unit when it is connected to suction.
    Significance: This bubbling indicates air leakage in the system. An air leak may be from the lung, insertion site, a loose connection in the drainage system, or a crack in the collection device.
    Nursing action: Determine the origin of the air leak. Use special clamps and begin by momentarily (no more than 10 seconds) clamping the chest tube, as close to the patient's chest as possible, and work your way down to the drainage unit. If the air leak at the drainage system is identified, the system needs to be replaced. Check all connections; make sure they are not loose. Use tape to reinforce connections. You should also assess the suction chamber for the proper fluid volume height, which controls the suction pressure. Replace water that has evaporated. Presence of GENTLE bubbling in the suction chamber is evidence that suction is being applied to the chest. Absence of bubbling indicates that there may be inadequate suction applied to the patient's chest. Suction may not be used; in this case, leave this chamber open to

atmospheric air (disconnect the suction regulator).

• Twelve hours after chest tube insertion, drainage stops from the chest tube.
Significance: A change from bloody to serous fluids indicates improvement. No drainage from the previous shift without any obvious cause (kinked tubes) indicates the lung has expanded.

Nursing action: Examine the patient's lungs, the chest tube site, and drainage system. Establish a baseline of vital signs, chest examination (auscultation, inspection, palpation, and percussion), and pain symptoms. The drainage tubing should be free of kinks and coiled on the bed for drainage into the system without dependent looping. The volume of fluid in the collection chamber is assessed to estimate the amount of fluid accumulated from the previous shift. Note the color, consistency, and any obvious odor (dark red to bright red color indicates bleeding). Report these findings to the physician for possible removal of the chest tube.

• Three days after insertion, drainage from the chest tube stops and there is no fluctuation in the fluid level with respiration. What is the significance of this?
Answer: There is a blockage or kink in the tubing.

• To apply suction to the suction chamber, at what level would you set the wall unit suction? What should you note in the suction chamber?
Answer: (-20 cm H20). Adequate fluid volume according to the physician's orders.

• If Mr. Davidson's chest tube became disconnected, what would you do? Are the appropriate instruments at the bedside?
Answer: Current practice is to quickly place the end of the chest tube in a container of sterile water or saline (such as the bottle kept at the bedside to replace the evaporated water in the suction chamber) until the entire drainage system can be replaced. Because of the risk of tension pneumothorax, clamping the tubing is not recommended. If the tube is pulled out of the patient's chest wall, immediately place an occlusive dressing (Vaseline gauze) over the site and notify the physician immediately.

• Which of the following is worse?
  • The chest tube becomes disconnected from the closed chest tube drainage system.
  • The closed chest tube drainage system becomes disconnected from the wall suction.
Answer: The chest tube becomes disconnected from the closed chest drainage system.

INDEX

Page numbers in **boldface type** indicate complete chapters.

AACN. *See* American Association of Colleges of Nursing
Academic advisement, **57–60**. *See also* Counseling
   by community college faculty, 20–21
   legal implications of, 60, 88, 89
   relationship to research and scholarship, 49
   as service, 53
Academic freedom
   loss of, 78
   U.S. Supreme Court statement on, 79
Academic Position Network (web site), 2
Academic requirements, changes in, 89
Academic year, 50, 178
Accreditation, 9, 23–24
   college–wide, 24
   of programs, 24
Accrediting organizations. *See also* Commission on
   Collegiate Nursing Education (CCNE); National
   League for Nursing Accreditation Commission
   (NLNAC)
   professional service with, 53
Ad hoc committees, 12, 53
Administrators, academic, titles and duties of, 10–11
Admission, of students with special needs, 104
Admissions office, 81
Advance organizers, 149
Advertising, of nursing faculty job positions, 6
Affective domain competency, evaluation of, 112, 113
Affirmative action cards, 2
Alcohol abuse, by students, 97
   academic advisement assistance for, 59
   case study of, 185–186
   policies for, 83, 84, 85
Alternative medicine, 144
ALT (newspaper), 66–67
American Academy of Nursing (AAN), 168
American Assembly of Men in Nursing (AAMN), 168
American Association of Colleges of Nursing (AACN),
   24, 168
   baccalaureate education guidelines of, 144–145
   curriculum development guidelines of, 142, 145
   job search database of, 2
   position statement on nursing scholarship of, 49
American Association of University Professors (AAUP)
   endorsement of "Statement of Principles on Academic
      Freedom and Tenure" by, 74
   faculty workload guidelines of, 62
American Association of University Women (AAUW),
   22–23
American Cancer Society, community service with, 54–55
American Journal of Nursing, 2
American Nurse, 2
American Nurses Association (ANA), 168, 169
   Code of Ethics of, 170
   collective bargaining role of, 174
   curriculum development guidelines of, 145
   faculty membership in, 170
   Nursing Agenda for Health Care Reform of, 173
   organizational restructuring of, 174
   political action by, 173
   Standards for Clinical Practice of, 170
   Standards of Clinical Nursing of, 171
   Strategic Action Team of, 173

American Organization of Nurse Executives (AONE), 168
Americans with Disabilities Act (ADA), 60
   reasonable accommodation requirement of, 30, 87, 104,
      105, 109, 110
   application to learning disabled students, 107–108
   inappropriate use of, 183–184
ANA. *See* American Nurses' Association
Anecdotal notes, 47, 110
Anxiety
   of new faculty, 177
   of students, about clinical performance, 44
Appeals. *See also* Grievance procedures; Hearings
   of grades, 36, 88, 97
   of tenure denial, 77–78
Apprenticeship, differentiated from mentoring, 68–69
Armed forces, nursing accreditation requirements of, 24
Assistive devices, for disabled students, 110
Associate degree programs
   comparison with baccalaureate programs, 144
   trends in, 145
Association of American Colleges (AAC), endorsement of
   "Statement of Principles on Academic Freedom and
   Tenure" by, 74
Association of Operating Room Nurses (AORN), 168
Attention deficit disorder (ADD), students with, 104,
   108–109
Attrition, of minority group students, 124
Audiovisual (AV) techniques and equipment
   use in classroom teaching, 25–26, 28
   use in distance education, 161, 162

Baccalaureate programs
   accreditation of, 24
   faculty workload in, 62–63
   goals of, 144
Behavior. *See also* Misconduct
   of faculty
      codes of, 20, 22
      at community colleges, 22
      policies for, 19–20, 81
      at senior colleges or universities, 19–20
      professional, influence on public attitudes toward nurses,
         170–171
   of students, disruptive, 31, 83
Belief systems, of students, 93–94
Black Issues in Education (web site), 2
Board of Nursing, web site of, 2
Board of regents, 11
Board of trustees, 11, 12
Book reviews, 75
Breast cancer, 54–55
Buckley Amendment. *See* Family Education Rights and
   Privacy Act (FERPA)
Bulletin boards, 138

Calendar, course, 27
Campus life, faculty involvement in, 20, 22–23
Cancellation, of classes, 88
Career counseling, for students with special physical needs,
   109, 110
Case–focused learning, 145
Case management, as curriculum component, 144

Case methods, for development of critical thinking, 42
Case sets, 149
Case studies, 31, **183–190**
   of academic dishonesty, 188–189
   use in classroom instruction, 28
   of development of critical thinking, 42
   of learning disabled students, 187–188
   of learning resource center instruction, 134, 189–190
   of maintenance of student standards, 183–184
   of research and scholarship activities, 184–185
   of student falsification of clinical records, 186–187
   of substance–abusing students, 185–186
CCNE. *See* Collegiate Commission for Nursing Education
Certification
   maintenance of, 181
   in nursing specialties, professional practice requirement
      of, 17
Chairpersons, of nursing units, 10
Chancellors, administrative duties of, 10
Cheating (academic dishonesty), 86–87
   case study of, 188–189
   by distance education students, 164
Chest tube drainage, learning resource center teaching
      module about, 189–190
Chief academic officers, 10, 11
Chief executive officers, 10–11
Chief nurse administrator, of nursing units, 9
Chronicle of Higher Education, nursing–related job
      advertisements in, 2
CINAHL (Cumulative Index to Nursing and Allied Health
      Literature), 136, 163
Civil Rights Acts, 60
Class
   cancellation of, 88
   student preparation for, 28, 98
Class assignments, cheating on, 86–87
   case study of, 188–189
   by distance education students, 164
Classroom, environment of, 25
Classroom teaching, **25–37**
   audiovisual equipment use in, 25–26, 28
   definition of, 25
   efficacy of, 31–32
   student participation in, 30–31
CLEP (College Level Examination Program), 59
Clinical Competence Rating Scale (CCRS), 118–121
Clinical courses. *See also* Clinical setting; Clinical
      teaching; Conferences, clinical; Laboratory courses
   community–based, 38, 39, 47
   distance education–based, 165
   students' failure of, 44, 47
Clinical pathways, 158
   lack of critical thinking in, 147–148
Clinical setting
   critical thinking evaluation in, 152–153
   pre– and post–conferences in, 15, 41, 45–46, 149–150
   psychomotor skills training in, 134
   student errors in, 43, 82–83, 87, 92
   student negligence in, 85
   student performance in
      evaluation of, 88, 112, 118
      effect of learning resource center practice on, 133
      poor, 96–97
      preparation work for, 98–99
   students' falsification of records in, 87
   team teaching in, 95–96
Clinical teaching, **38–48**
   evaluation of, 65

Clinical teaching *(cont.)*
   faculty workload in, 62
   instructor's responsibility in, 38
   by new faculty, 16
   patient selection in, 39–40
   relationship with clinical staff in, 38, 39, 41, 45–46
   student supervision in, 41–42, 47
Clinical Teaching Evaluation (CTE), 65
Clinics, faculty–run, 17
Clinton, Bill, 173
Codes of behavior, for faculty, 20, 22
Codes of ethics, 81, 168, 173
Cognitive skills training, 131
Colleagues. *See also* Peer review
   support of, 181
Collective bargaining, 174
College(s), differentiated from universities, 9
College Level Examination Program (CLEP), 59
College of nursing, definition of, 9
Colleges and universities
   Carnegie classification of, 14
   goals of, 9, 13
   governance of, 11
      participatory, 13
   public differentiated from private, 11–12
   secular differentiated from nonsecular, 12
Commission on Collegiate Nursing Education (CCNE), 9
   nursing program accreditation by, 24
   site visitors for, 53
Committees
   ad hoc, 12, 53
   role in colleges and universities, 12–13
   search, 2, 5–8
   tenure, 76
Committee work, 56
   by community college faculty, 22–23
   by senior college or university faculty, 15, 19
   on tenure committees, 76
Communication
   asynchronous, 161, 162, 166
   faculty–student, 92–93
      with nonnative English speakers, 94–95
   synchronous, 161, 162, 166
Communication skills training, 131, 132
Community colleges. *See also* Associate degree programs
   faculty roles in, 20–24
Community groups, faculty's participation in, 16–17
Competence
   clinical, of students, 35, 40
      evaluation of, 118–121
      evolution of, 118
   of faculty, 17, 26
Computer(s). *See also* Internet
   integration into the classroom, **136–139**
Computer–based distance education, 161, 162, 163–164,
      166, 167
Computer–based examinations, 115
Computer–based practice examinations, 99–100
Concept mapping, 94, 157
Conferences, clinical
   post–, 15, 41, 45–46, 149–150
   pre–, 15, 41
Confidentiality
   of faculty evaluation by students, 65, 66–67
   of patient records, 82
   of student information and records, 60, 81–82
Conflict resolution, gender or cultural, 123–124
Consulting, as service activity, 54, 56

Content maps, use in curriculum development, 143
Continuing education, critical thinking training in, 150
Continuous quality management (CQM), 67
Contracts
    with clinical agencies, 38
    of faculty
        for academic year, 178
        union negotiation of, 22, 23
        teaching–learning, 98
Coping strategies, 181
Copyright Act, 164
Copyright issues, in distance education, 164–165
Correction, of students, 92–93
Correspondence courses, 161, 162
Counseling, 90–91
    for clinical performance–related anxiety, 44
    of disruptive students, 31
Course calendar, 27
Course development, workload credit for, 178
Course load, of students, 155–156
Credit hours, of courses, 155–156
Crisis counseling, 90
Critical thinking, **147–154,** 171
    definition of, 147
    evaluation of, 150–154
    in professional and political activities, 173–174
    students' lack of, 45
    teaching of, 29, 147–150
        in clinical setting, 42–43
        use of computers in, 138
        in learning resource center instruction, 134
Critical thinking log, 98–99
CTE (Clinical Teaching Evaluation), 65
Cultural brokerage, 124
Cultural conflict resolution, 123–124
Cultural customs, of students, 93–94
Cultural issues. *See also* English as a second language
        (ESL); Language(s)
    in the curriculum, 124–125, 144
    evaluation of international students, 112
    teaching diverse student groups, 93–94, **123–129**
Culture, institutional, 22
Culture shock, 127
Cumulative Index to Nursing and Allied Health Literature
        (CINAHL), 136, 163
Curriculum
    core, 142
    cultural diversity themes within, 124–125, 144
    definition of, 140
    development of, **140–145**
        by community college faculty, 21
        content maps in, 143
        guidelines for, 142
        objectives in, 143
        trends in, 144–145
    "null," 147
Curriculum vitae, 1, 3

Date rape victims, academic advisement assistance for, 59
Deans
    of the faculty, 11
    of nursing programs, 180
    of nursing units, 9, 10
Debates, 28, 31
Decision–making, in governance of academic institutions,
        13
Defamation, of students, 89
Delta Pi, 169

Departments, academic, 9. *See also* Nursing departments
Dependency, of students, 91
Digital Millennium Copyright Act, 164
Directors, of nursing units, 9
Disability, discrimination based on, legislative prohibition
        of, 60, 104–105. *See also* Americans with Disabilities
        Act (ADA)
Disabled students, 102, 104–111
    academic advisement for, 59
    assistive devices for, 110
    with attention deficit disorder, 104, 108–109
    learning disabled, 102, 104, 106–108, 187–188
    legal responsibilities to, 87
    with special physical needs, 104, 109–110
Disadvantaged (challenged) students, 102–104
Disciplinary actions
    for student substance abuse, 83
    for students' unsafe clinical practices, 44
Discrimination
    implication for academic advisement, 60
    toward disabled persons, legislative prohibition of, 60,
        104–105. *See also* Americans with Disabilities Act
        (ADA)
Discussions, by students, 28, 30–31
Dishonesty, academic, 86–87
    case study of, 188–189
    by distance education students, 164
Disruptive students, 31, 83
Distance education, **161–167**
    comparison with traditional education, 161–162
    copyright issues in, 164–165
    course development in, 163–164
    types of, 162
Doctoral degree
    faculty members' lack of, 74, 75
    as tenure qualification, 75
Doctoral degree programs
    accreditation of, 24
    research mentors in, 72
Domains of Practice (Benner), 158, 159, 171
Domestic violence victims, academic advisement assistance
        for, 59
Dress, of faculty members, 20
Drug abuse, by students, 97
    case study of, 185–186
    policies for, 83, 84, 85
Drug abusing students, academic advisement assistance for,
        59
Drug testing, random, 83
Due process
    constitutional basis for, 60
    procedural and substantive, 85–86

Eastern Nursing Research Society, 169
Education Amendments of 1972, 60
Electronic mail (e–mail), 138
English as a second language (ESL), 94–95
    of disadvantaged (challenged) students, 102, 103
Environmental issues, in the curriculum, 144
Equipment. *See also* Computer(s)
    audiovisual (AV), 25–26, 28, 161, 162
    in clinical setting, 45
Errors
    in academic advisement, 59
    by students
        clarification of, 29
        in clinical setting, 43, 82–83, 87, 92, 108, 187–188
        in medication administration, 43, 108, 187–188

Essay questions, 32, 113, 114
  advantages and disadvantages of, 114
  grading of, 116
Ethical issues. *See* Legal and ethical issues
Evaluation. *See also* Grades; Grading; Grading policies;
    Examinations
  of candidates for tenure, 76–77
  of clinical skills
    of disabled students, 110
    of distance education students, 165
    self–evaluation of, 96
    written assignments for, 158–159
  of critical thinking ability, 150–154
  of curriculum, 145
  of distance education courses, 166
  of faculty, **64–67**
    in clinical teaching, 65
    formative *versus* summative, 66
    latest trends in, 66–67
    by peers, 64, 65, 180
    by students, 36–37, 179–180
    of tenured faculty, 79
  measurement issues in, 117–118
  self–evaluation
    by faculty, 64–65
    of students' clinical performance, 96
  by students
    of faculty, 36–37, 179–180
    self–evaluation, 96
  of students, 29, 31–32
    of clinical performance, 96, 110, 158–159, 165
    feedback in, 19
    of learning disabled students, 106
    legal implications of, 88
    by new faculty, 179
    of psychomotor skills, 112, 121
    of students with special needs, 110
  of technology–assisted learning, 139
  of transcultural teaching methods, 125–126
  of web sites, 136–137
Evidence–based practice, 145
Examinations
  cheating on, 86–87
  clinical, 88, 118
    preparation work for, 98–99
  computer–assisted, 99–100, 115, 138
  construction of, 15, 32–33, 112–114
  use in critical thinking evaluations, 151–152, 154
  dates of, 27
  for disabled students, 105
    case study of, 183–184
  for distance education students, 164, 166
  item analysis of, 114–115
  for learning disabled students, 107, 108
  for nonnative English–speaking students, 94–95
  post–grading class review of, 33–34
  reuse of, 115
  students' failure of, by an excessive number of students,
      33
  types of questions
    advantages and disadvantages of, 114
    essays, 32, 113, 114, 116
    fill–in–the–blanks, 32, 114
    matching, 32, 114
    multiple–choice, 32, 112, 113, 115–116, 151
    true/false, 32, 114
  validity and reliability of, 117, 118–119
Expert witnesses, 56

Extra–work activities, 16–17

Faculty
  decision–making authority of, 13
  inconsistency of, 88, 96
  minority–group, 104
  new
    anxiety of, 177
    mentoring of, **68–73**, 184, 185
    perspectives from, **177–182**
    stressors of, 177–178
    teaching assignments of, 16
    transition from clinical practice by, 177
    workload of, 22
  nondoctoral, 74, 75
  part–time, 23, 74
  physical appearance of, 20, 170–171
  roles of, **14–24.** *See also* Research; Service; Teaching
    in community colleges, 20–24
    as "sacred triad," 14
    in senior colleges and universities, 14–20
Faculty positions
  acquisition of, **1–8**
  nontenure track, 74–75
Faculty rank, as job interview issue, 4
Faculty senate, 12–13
Faculty–student relationship, 91
  in classroom instruction, 28–29
  in distance education, 165, 166
  in learning resource centers, 134
  in student organizations, 20
Faculty wives' clubs, 22–23
Failure, 96–97
  in clinical courses, 44, 47
  by an excessive number of students, 33
  as indicator of teacher's competence, 35–36
Family Education Rights and Privacy Act (FERPA), 60,
    81–82, 110
Filing systems, 18–19
Fill–in–the–blanks questions, 32
  advantages and disadvantages of, 114
Funding, of research, 15–16, 52

Gatekeeping responsibility, of nursing faculty, 112
Gender conflict resolution, 123–124
Gifts, from students, 82
Goals, of colleges and universities, 9, 13
Governance, of colleges and universities, 11
  participatory, 13
Grades
  calculation of, 34–35
  curving of, 35
  failing, 96–97
    in clinical courses, 44, 47
    of an excessive number of students, 33
    as indicator of teachers' competence, 35–36
  student appeals of, 36, 88, 97
Grading
  of clinical performance, 46–47, 159
  of critical thinking activities, 153
  of nonnative English–speaking students, 94
  of psychomotor skills, 132
  of short answer and essay questions, 116
  of written assignments, 34
Grading policies, 97
  legal implications of, 81, 83, 88
Graduate students, academic advisement for, 58
Graduation requirements, legal implications of, 88, 89

Grants, for research, 15–16
Grant writing, workload credits for, 178
Grievance procedures, 20
    for grade appeals, 36
    for tenure denial, 77–78

Handbooks
    faculty, 19–20
    student, 20, 84
Health care policy, faculty and student influence on, 172
Health care reform, 173
Health care system, improvement of, 172
Hearings. *See also* Grievance procedures
    for student policy violations, 84
        due process in, 85–86
Henshaw, Chris, 14
Homework, 27–28, 32
Honor organizations, 16, 22–23, 168, 169

Injuries, to patients, by students, 82–83
International Council of Nurses (ICN), 168, 169, 174
    Code of Ethics of, 81
International health issues, in the curriculum, 144
International students, evaluation of, 112
Internet
    advertising of faculty positions on, 6
    use in the classroom, 137–138
    copyright information web sites on, 164–165
    cultural diversity web sites on, 128
    distance education web sites on, 161, 162
    faculty evaluation web sites on, 66–67
Interviews
    in critical thinking evaluations, 154
    of nursing faculty job applicants, 3–4
        illegal questions in, 4
        on–site, 3–4, 6
        by telephone, 3, 4, 5, 6

Job descriptions, of nursing faculty positions, 5–6
Job search, for nursing faculty positions, 1–5
Joint appointments, 18
Joint Commission on Accreditation of Healthcare
    Organizations (JCAHO), professional competence
    guidelines of, 17
Journaling, by culturally diverse students, 125
Journal of Nursing Scholarship, 2
Journals
    authorship fees of, 51–52
    use in clinical evaluation, 159
    use in critical thinking evaluation, 154
    nonrefereed, 75
    refereed, 51, 75

King, Martin Luther, Jr., 124
(Susan G.) Komen Foundation, New York "Race for the
    Cure," 54–55

Laboratory courses
    teaching hours in, 18
    workloads of, 155–156
Language(s). *See also* English as a second language (ESL)
    of nonnative English speakers, 94–95
    of students, faculty's proficiency in, 126
Language skills, of students, 94–95
    deficiencies in
        of disadvantaged (challenged) students, 102, 103
        of learning disabled students, 106, 107
Lawsuits, 82, 83–84

Leadership
    among minority group students, 124
    of professional organizations, 75, 76
Learning
    active, 28, 130
    case–focused, 145
    in distance education, 161–162
    passive, 28
    problem–focused, 145
Learning curve, in distance education, 166
Learning disabled students, 102, 104, 106–108
    case study of, 187–188
Learning environment, 43
    for students with special needs, 110–111
Learning resource centers (LRCs), **130–135**
    case studies of, 134, 189–190
    instructors/coordinators of, 130, 131, 132, 133, 134
Learning styles, 94
Lecture method, 29–30
    for critical thinking development, 149
Lecture notes, students' copies of, 30
Legal and ethical issues, **81–89**
    academic advisement, 60, 88, 89
    anecdotal notes, 47, 110
    as curriculum topic, 100
    disabled students, 87, 104–105, 110
    faculty qualifications and responsibilities, 181
    grading policies, 81, 83, 88
    legal rights of nurses, 173–174
    validity and reliability of measurement instruments, 118
Legal council, for colleges and universities, 81
Letters
    of recommendation/reference, 58
        for academically weak students, 59–60
        legal and ethical responsibilities for, 86
    for tenure application, 76–77
Library, distance education students' access to, 163–164
Lifestyles, of students, 93–94
Linear thinking, in nursing process, 148
Literature searching, online, 136–137, 163–164
Lobbying, 172, 174–175

Malpractice
    educational, 83–84
    medical, 82
Marketing, of distance education courses, 164
Master's degree programs, accreditation of, 24
Matching questions, 32
    advantages and disadvantages of, 114
Mathematical skills, of learning disabled students, 107, 108
Medical procedures, performance by students, 82
Medication administration
    errors in, 43, 108, 187–188
    by learning disabled students, 108
    timing and supervision of, 40
MEDLINE, 136, 163
Mentally ill students, academic advisement assistance for,
    59
Mentor, differentiated from preceptor, master, or role
    model, 68–69
Mentoring, 53, 169
    definition of, 68
    in doctoral research, 72
    of faculty, 90–91
    of new faculty, **68–73**
        case studies of, 184, 185
        disadvantages of, 71
    of tenure candidates, 77

Merit guidelines, 19
Minority group students. *See also* Cultural issues;
    Disadvantaged (challenged) students
  leadership and mentoring of, 124
Misconduct
  of faculty, 20
  of students. *See also* Alcohol abuse; Drug abuse;
      Substance abuse
    academic dishonesty, 86–87, 164, 188–189
    falsification of clinical records, 87, 186–187
Mission
  institutional, 9, 14, 140–141
  of nursing programs, 140, 141
Montag, Mildred, 144
Multiple–choice questions, 32, 113
  advantages and disadvantages of, 114
  international students' unfamiliarity with, 112
  for measurement of critical thinking, 151
  simplicity of, 115–116

Narratives, use in critical thinking evaluations, 154
National Association of Profile Nurses (NAPN), 168
National Black Nurses Association (NBNA), 168
National Council Licensure Examination (NCLEX)
  multiple–choice format of, 32, 99
  performance on, effect of learning resource center
      practice on, 133
  student preparation for, 99–100, 115
National Education Association (NEA), Code of Ethics of,
    81
National League for Nursing Accreditation Commission
    (NLNAC), 24
  site visitors for, 53
National League for Nursing (NLN), 24, 168
  curriculum development guidelines of, 142, 145
  faculty membership in, 170
  Nursing Agenda for Health Care Reform of, 173
National Organization of Nurse Practitioner Faculty
    (NONPF), 168
National Student Nurses Association (NSNA), 55, 168
  web site of, 137
NCLEX. *See* National Council Licensure Examination
NetMeeting, 166
Networking
  by minority group students, 124
  by search committees, 6
New York State Nurses Association, Capital District #9
    local, 169
Nightingale, Florence, 53
Nontenure track positions, 74–75
Notecards
  use in clinical learning activities, 158
  use with reading assignments, 156–157
Notes, anecdotal, 47, 110
Note–taking, for clinical examinations, 99–100
Nurse managers
  as evaluators of faculty clinical instruction skills, 65
  relationship with faculty, 16
Nurse practice acts, 168, 173
Nurses in AIDS Care (NAC), 168
Nursing care plans
  as assignment, 158
  lack of critical thinking in, 147–148
Nursing departments
  definition of, 9
  new faculty members' orientation to, 180–181
Nursing division, definition of, 9

Nursing League for Nursing Accrediting Commission
    (NLNAC)
  accreditation standards of, 9
  site visitors for, 53
Nursing process, lack of critical thinking in, 147
Nursing profession
  ethnic and racial composition of, 126–127
  public attitudes toward, 170–171
Nursing programs
  administrators of, 10
  mission of, 140, 141
  organizational structure of, 9, 10
Nursing's Agenda for Health Care Reform, 173
Nursing Standards of Care, 168
Nursing units, within colleges or universities, 9

Observation instruments, use in critical thinking evaluation,
    154
Office hours, of community college faculty, 20
Office of Students with Disabilities, 59
"One Minute Manager," 159
One–minute papers, 29, 32
Organizational structure, **9–13**
Orientation
  of new faculty, 180–181
  of students
    to clinical agencies, 39
    of disadvantaged (challenged) students, 104

Parents, of students
  meetings with academic advisors, 58
  release of student information to, 81–82
Part–time faculty, 74
  union membership of, 23
Patient care management, senior students' preparation for,
    100
Patients, injuries to, by students, 82–83
Patient selection, for clinical instruction, 39–40
Peer counseling, for minority group students, 124
Peer review
  of faculty, 64, 65, 180
  of journal articles or presentations, 51, 75
  of research proposals, 52
  of tenure applications, 76
Personal problems, of students, 90
Phi Kappa Phi, 22–23
Philippine Nurses Association of America (PNAA), 168
Philosophy
  institutional,17
  of nursing programs, 140
  personal, 17
  professional, 1
Photocopying, of medical records, by students, 82
Physical appearance
  of faculty, 20, 170–171
  of students, 170–171
Policies
  for faculty behavior, 19–20, 81
  student
    for grade review appeals, 36, 81, 83, 88
    institutional, 84
    nursing–specific, 84–85, 87
    for substance abuse, 83, 84, 85, 97–98
Political action committees (PACs), 173
Political education, 171–175
Political influence, of professional organizations, 169
Political organizations, 169

Portfolios
    use in critical thinking evaluations, 154
Portfolios *(cont.)*
    teaching, 66
Post–conference, clinical, 15, 41, 45–46, 149–150
Postdoctoral programs, research mentors in, 72
Post–tenure review, 79
PowerPoint, 2
Practice
    by community college faculty, 21
    domains of, 158, 159, 171
    evidence–based, 145
    by senior college or university faculty, 17–18
Practice acts, 168, 173
Preceptors, 18
    differentiated from mentor, master, or role model, 68–69
    for distance education students, 165, 167
Pre–conference, clinical, 15, 41
Preparation
    by faculty, for classroom teaching, 178
    by students
        for class, 28, 98
        for clinical courses, 98–99
        for multiple–choice examinations, 99–100
        for National Council Licensure Examination
            (NCLEX), 99–100, 115
Presentations
    at conferences, as tenure qualification, 75
    by distance education students, 166
    during job interviews, 3
    refereed, 51
    software use in, 137
Presidents, of colleges or universities, 10–11
Probationary period, for faculty, 75
Problem–focused learning, 145
Problem–solving, 31
    evaluation of, 120
    in learning resource center instruction, 134
    in professional and political activities, 173–174
Professional development, institutional policies for, 181
Professional organizations, 168–171. *See also names of*
        individual organizations
    categories of, 168–169
    faculty participation in, 16, 169–170
    leadership roles in, 75, 76
Professional practice interests, 173–174
Promotion
    relationship to time spent in scholarly activities, 50
    requirements for, 19, 52, 177
Provost, administrative duties of, 10, 11
Psychomotor skills, evaluation of, 112, 121
Psychomotor skills training
    in clinical setting, 40
    in learning resource centers, 130, 131–132, 133–134
Publications
    of faculty, 50–52
    single–authored, 51
Public attitudes, toward nurses, 170–171
"Publish or perish," 52

Question asking
    by faculty, as Socratic approach, 150
    by students, 29–30, 43, 44–45, 92–93
Questionnaires, use in critical thinking evaluations, 154
Quota system, for tenure, 78

Reading assignments, 27, 28
    completion of, 156

Reading assignments *(cont.)*
    notecard responses to, 156–157
Reading skill deficiencies, of learning disabled students,
        106, 107
Reality shock, experienced by new faculty members,
        177–178
Reappointment, of faculty, 177
Records
    for academic advisement, 58
    clinical
        falsification by students, 87, 186–187
        photocopying by students, 82
    of students, 60, 81–82
Recruitment, of minority group students, 126–127
References, for nursing faculty job applicants, 1, 2
Referrals, to counseling services, 90
Regents, board of, 11
Registered Care Technologist (RCT) proposal, 173
Registered nurse completion students, academic
        advisement for, 59
Registrar's office, 81
Rehabilitation Act of 1973, 60, 104, 105
Reminder files, 19
Research, 49–52. *See also* Publications; Scholarship
    cost of, 52
    definition of, 49
    differentiated from scholarship, 49
    as faculty role, 14, 15
    funding of, 15–16, 52
    mentoring in, 72, 185
    student involvement in, 19
    time scheduling for, 50, 184–185
    workload credits for, 178
Research proposals, peer review of, 52
Résumés, 1, 3
Retention, of minority group students, 125, 126
Risk management reports, 82–83
Role(s), of faculty. *See also* Research; Service; Teaching
    comparison with non–nursing faculty, 21
    outside the work setting, 16–17
    "sacred triad" of, 14
Role models
    differentiated from mentors, preceptors, or masters,
        68–69
    disadvantaged (challenged) students' lack of, 102, 103
    faculty as, 53, 170
    tenured faculty as, 77
Role playing, by students, 28, 30–31
Roy's Adaptation Model, of research, 49

"Sacred triad," of faculty roles, 14
Salaries
    as job interview issue, 4
    in joint appointments, 18
Scholarship, 49–52
    differentiated from research, 49
    as faculty role, 14, 15
    mentoring in, 185
    as tenure qualification, 75
    time scheduling for, 184, 185
        effect of faculty workload on, 62–63
School of nursing, definition of, 9
Search committees, 2, 5–8
Self–confidence, low, of students, 92
Self–esteem, low, of disabled students, 105
Self–evaluation
    by faculty, 64–65

Self–evaluation *(cont.)*
  of students' clinical performance, 96
Senate, faculty, 12–13
Senior students, preparation for patient care management
    role, 100
Service, 20, 22, **53–56**
  to the college or university, 53. *See also* Committee work
  community, 54–55
    by students, 172
    as tenure qualification, 75–76
  definition of, 53
  as faculty role, 14, 17, 53
    relationship to research and scholarship, 49
  professional, 53
  as tenure requirement, 55
  time scheduling for, 50, 62–63
Sigma Theta Tau Honor Society of Nursing, 168
  research funding by, 16
Simulations, use in critical thinking evaluations, 154
Skill enhancement, by faculty, 179
Skill maintenance, by faculty, 17
Skills laboratory. *See* Learning resource centers (LRCs)
Socialization
  of distance education students, 165–166
  of new faculty. *See* Mentoring, of new faculty
  of new graduates, 100
  of students, 170
Social relationships
  of distance education students, 165–166
  faculty–student. *See* Faculty–student relationship
  of minority group students, 124
Social skills, of learning disabled students, 107
Socratic approach, 150
Software, use in presentations, 137
Special needs students, **102–111**
  academic advisement for, 59
  disabled students, 102, 104–111
    with attention deficit disorder (ADD), 104, 108–109
    evaluation of, 110
    learning disabled, 102, 104, 106–108, 187–188
    with special physical needs, 104, 109–110
  disadvantaged (challenged) students, 102–104
  identification of, 102
  learning environment for, 110–111
Staff
  of clinical settings, 38, 39, 41, 45–46
    patient care by, 45
  of learning resource centers, 134–135
Staff development, critical thinking training in, 150
Standards of care, 168
Standards of practice, 170, 173
State attorney general's office, 81
"Statement of Principles on Academic Freedom and
    Tenure," 74, 75
State nurse associations
  collective bargaining by, 174
  research funding by, 16
Stokes, Elizabeth, 14
Stressors, of new faculty, 177–178
Student advisement. *See* Academic advisement
Student interaction. *See also* Social relationships
  by distance education students, 165–166
Student nurse associations, 55, 168
  minority group students' participation in, 124
  web site of, 137
Student organizations
  disadvantaged (challenged) students' participation in,
    104

Student organizations *(cont.)*
  faculty advisors for, 53
Students. *See also* Special needs students
  academically marginal, 35–36
Students *(cont.)*
  concerns of and about, **90–101**
  cultural diversity of, 93–94, **123–129**
  dependent, 91
  educational malpractice lawsuits by, 83–84
  faculty evaluation by, 36–37, 64, 65, 66–67
  performance of medical procedures by, 82
  physical appearance of, 170–171
  question asking by, 29–30, 43, 44–45, 92–93
  release of information about, 60, 81–82
  "working on faculty members'" license by, 82
Substance abuse
  disciplinary actions for, 83
  by students, 97
Substance abuse policies, 97–98
Supervisors, faculty evaluation by, 64
Support groups
  faculty's participation in, 17
  for minority group students, 124
Suspension, of students, for unsafe clinical practices, 44
Syllabus, 26, 83
Syllabus guides, 81

Tape recording, of lectures, 30
Task forces, 53
Teaching
  evaluation of. *See* Evaluation, of faculty
  as faculty role, 14, 179
    priority of, 19
    relationship to professional practice, 18
    relationship to research and scholarship, 49, 50
    in senior colleges or universities, 14–15
Teaching assignments, 16
  of community college faculty, 23
  comparison with non–nursing faculty, 18
Teaching load. *See also* Workload
  calculation of, 178
  consistency of, 179
  differentiated from workload, 61
Teaching methods
  for classroom teaching, 28–31
  for culturally diverse students, 125–126
  for disabled students, 105–106, 110–111
    for learning disabled students, 107–108
    for students with attention deficit disorder, 109
    for students with special physical needs, 109–110
  Socratic approach, 150
  trends in, 145
Teaching portfolio, 66
Teaching resource files, 18–19
Teaching styles, differences in, 96
Team teaching, 16, 95–96
Technical support, for distance education, 166–167
Technology integration, in the classroom, **136–139**
Tenure, 74–79
  definition of, 74
  denial of, 77–78
  opposition to, 78–79
  purpose and benefits of, 74
  quota system for, 78
  relationship to time spent in scholarly activities, 50
  requirements for, 19, 22, 52, 55, 75–76, 177
    effect of faculty workload on, 63
Tenure files, 77

Tests. *See* Examinations
Textbook publishers, test banks of, 16, 115
Textbooks, 26–27
  for distance education, 163
Theory, application to practice, 121
Therapists, faculty as, 90, 91
Time scheduling
  of academic advisement, 50
  of assignments, 32
  of classroom teaching, 27–28, 178
  of clinical teaching, 42, 43
  by community college faculty, 22
  of examinations, 32
  by new faculty members, 177
  of research and scholarly activities, 50, 184–185
  by senior college or university faculty, 19
  of service activities, 55
  of work week, 15
Total quality management (TQM), 67
Transcripts, of job applicants, 2
Transcultural concepts. *See* Cultural issues
Transfer students
  academic advisement for, 59
  orientation programs for, 104
Triangulation, use in critical thinking evaluations, 153–154
True–false questions, 32
  advantages and disadvantages of, 114
Trustees, board of, 11, 12
Tuition rates, 12

Unions
  faculty, 22, 23
  nurses' membership in, 174
U.S. Constitution, 60

U.S. Department of Education, 24
U.S. Supreme Court, statement on academic freedom, 79
Universities. *See also* Colleges and universities
  differentiated from colleges, 9
Unsafe clinical practices, of students, 44. *See also* Errors, by students

Vice president for academic affairs, 10, 11
Volunteering, by faculty. *See* Service

Web sites. *See also specific web sites*
  evaluation of, 136–137
  of faculty, 138
  use in job searches, 2
Workload, **61–63**
  calculation of, 61–62
  of community college faculty, 20
  comparison with non–nursing faculty workload, 63
  definition of, 61
  in distance education, 96, 166
  in research and scholarship, 50
  of senior college or university faculty,15
Work organization
  by community college faculty, 21
  by senior college or university faculty, 18–19
Work week, scheduling of, 15
Written assignments, **155–160**
  in clinical instruction, 42, 158–159
  for development of critical thinking, 42, 153
  for evaluation of students' achievement, 117
  grading of, 34
  time requirements for, 155–156

Year, academic, 50, 178